DANCING DEEPER STILL

THE PRACTICE OF CONTACT IMPROVISATION

MARTIN KEOGH

INTIMATELY ROOTED BOOKS

Terra Incognita

*There are vast realms of consciousness still undreamed
      of*
*vast ranges of experience, like the humming of unseen
      harps,*
we know nothing of, within us.

*Oh when man has escaped from the barbed-wire
      entanglement*
of his own ideas and his own mechanical devices
*there is a marvelous rich world of contact and sheer
      fluid beauty*
and fearless face-to-face awareness of now-naked life
and me, and you, and other men and women
*and grapes, and ghouls, and ghosts and green
      moonlight*
and ruddy-orange limbs stirring the limbo
of the unknown air, and eyes so soft
softer than the space between the stars,
and all things, and nothing, and being and not-being
alternately palpitant,
when at last we escape the barbed-wire enclosure
of Know Thyself, knowing we can never know,
*we can but touch, and wonder, and ponder, and make
      our effort*
and dangle in a last fastidious fine delight
as the fuchsia does, dangling her reckless drop
of purple after so much putting forth
and slow mounting marvel of a little tree.

– D.H. Lawrence

Dancing Deeper Still
The Practice of Contact Improvisation
Intimately Rooted Books
©2018 Martin Keogh. All rights reserved

ISBN-978-1-7752430-1-4 (Hardcover)
ISBN-978-1-7752430-4-5 (Paperback)
ISBN-978-1-7752430-3-8 (Ebook)

Cover design: Elizabeth Mackey
Front cover photo: Sören Wacker: sorenwacker.pixieset.com
Dancers: Rose Leighton and Jeanette Soria
Back cover dance photo: Thomas Häntzchel
Dancers: Martin Keogh and Rick Nodine
Back cover bio photo: Nadja Meister

Many essays in this book first appeared
in Contact Quarterly, Proximity, and Yes! Magazine

Dancing Deeper Still: Version X (2018)
Former Editions:
The Earth is Breathing You (2001)
The Art of Waiting (2003)

Get in touch:
contact@martinkeogh.com

ALSO BY MARTIN KEOGH

Hope Beneath Our Feet

Restoring Our Place in the Natural World

As Much Time as it Takes

Handbook for the Bereaved, their Family and Friends

Etched in Your Brain Name Games

How To Guide for Teachers, Group Facilitators

and Insightful Leaders Everywhere

Book information, videos, and workshop itinerary:

martinkeogh.com

This book is dedicated to

Dylan Keogh

CONTENTS

INTRODUCTION

For decades I dreamt of becoming an author. I imagined myself in a sparsely furnished cabin with a well-tended fire, writing for hours each day. Yet, that dream lacked one important detail. Whenever I sat down to write I became flummoxed in my hunt for subject matter.

Then 9/11 came crashing into our lives. Within a week of that event I realized I did not need to go on some wild pursuit; my subject would be Contact Improvisation (C.I.), the dance form I spent so many decades teaching and performing. In between touring and parenting and partnering, I began to write.

The San Francisco, Bay Area has long had a thriving community of Contact dancers. My decades there provided me with a wealth of learning. We danced together at weekly Contact jams, at residential dancing events, and at rehearsals and 'labs' to research the form. We also danced in city parks, in the downtown financial district, and at 'dune diving' parties at Point Reyes National Seashore. During one trip to the zoo we marked off an area of grass with rope, put up an official-looking sign that proclaimed, "New at the Zoo," and a group of us had a round robin of dances in the enclosure. People stopped and read the sign. Some looked at us quizzically. A few joined in.

After a day of dancing on Limantour Beach, a group sat around a campfire listening to the waves breaking on the shore. A few of us were part of Touchdown Dance, an organization that introduces Contact Improvisation to the blind. As we sat surrounded by darkness, watching the dance of flames and the shimmering coals, one person asked, "How would you describe fire to a blind person?" Our attempts to create a verbal picture that gave the sense of fire were feeble next to the crackling and prancing of the flames that warmed us. How do you describe something as varied and changeable as fire without putting a person's hand in it? In that moment I realized why it's hard to define Contact Improvisation. Like fire, it's in motion, it's mercurial. The essays in this book are my attempt to describe the crackle and blaze of our dancing.

One of the more challenging aspects of researching Contact Improvisation, because this extemporaneous form calls for an ongoing inquiry, is the constant admission that I don't have it all figured out... and I never will. These essays catch me at moments in the investigation. They reflect questions and answers that illuminate an instant rather than a doctrine. In writing, I find the same challenge as when I dance or teach, to enter a sense of improvisational inquiry rather than a set of dogmatic rules. Every person has their own individual doorways into the dance. These are some of my doorways - what I've experienced and learned after almost forty years of engaging this form as a teacher and performer.

In a large dance complex in Oakland, California I saw two

modern dance teachers peering at a Contact class through a small window in the door to the studio. I overheard one say to the other, "I can't believe it, they're sitting and talking again."

What she found so perplexing is something I cherish about the form. This dance puts a priority on our ability to be lucid in the moment, and our capacity to articulate our experience and research to others. This has helped my writing.

I enter the writing in the same way I warm up for dancing. I'm not climbing a mountain; it's not some Herculean task. I don't need to rise to the occasion. I descend into that place in myself where I am already prepared to dance, where the language is already present.

Language is important. How do we track down those metaphors that give a visceral feeling for what we do when we dance? My job is to tame a few of the many thoughts. To entice, coax, and persuade images to sit on the page.

The hardest images to catch are the nocturnal ones, with their reflective eyes that can only be glimpsed at night. How does one write about the shadow side of the dance, the ephemeral qualities of the form, the dance of boundaries and emotion, the confluence with the spiritual, the rapture? For those images to be seen in all their feral wonder, one has to enter without a light and magnify other senses to perceive what is present.

I'm fortunate to have a passion for both dancing and language. Written during four decades of rapport and grappling, of discord and harmony, this book is my love letter to the dance. What follows is a series of essays, collaborative writings, and teaching research notes. You can read this book from the beginning or you can thumb through the pages and start reading when whim moves you.

I am grateful to Steve Paxton for his initial outlandish idea to gather a group of people to investigate his ideas that became C.I. My appreciation goes to the originators for their foresight to not codify the dance and become the "C.I. police." This allowed Contact Improvisation to grow organically so it could mature into something that no one could have intended or even imagined.

I'm thankful for the generosity of all my teachers, and to Nancy Stark Smith for her commitment to language and her decades of cultivating the form through the Contact Quarterly magazine. Most of all, thanks to my students, collaborators, and dance partners that continue to make life so rich.

I also dedicate this book to you, the reader. Parts were written in San Miguel de Allende in the high desert in Mexico. Sitting outside at a cast iron table, surrounded by purple and crimson bougainvillea blossoms, visiting hummingbirds and the sounds of bells and chickens. The colors of the sidewalk flagstones after a rain, the smell of roasted poblano chilies filled with cheese, the cooing of doves feed my desire to colorfully bring this dance into language. And parts of this book were written in the temperate rain forest by the Salish Sea in the company of seals, river otters and orcas. They swim through these pages. In reading these essays I hope that you receive some of the pleasure I experienced in writing them.

PART I

THE TIME OF YOUR LIFE

Recently I returned to the Southeast to teach a two-weekend Contact Improvisation workshop in Washington, D.C. and Richmond, Virginia. I've taught in these communities several times before and didn't want to repeat my tried-and-true material. To challenge myself and the students, I created a theme I needed to grow into. The workshop was titled "The Time of Your Life". This was the description:

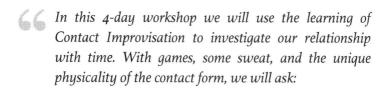 *In this 4-day workshop we will use the learning of Contact Improvisation to investigate our relationship with time. With games, some sweat, and the unique physicality of the contact form, we will ask:*

- *How do we relate to having only a finite amount of time?*
- *What does it mean to have "enough" time?*
- *How can we dilate time by putting our attention in the details?*

These questions will arise as we master more of the skills and thrills of the Contact form. Special emphasis on surprising ourselves in flight and extended follow-through.

I was interested to delve into experiencing time passing in a way that was kinesthetic rather than conceptual. My goal was to keep our explorations experiential and based in sensation. I wanted to see, when we dilated our attention to notice the details of each moment, if time would slow down.

I've always been interested in time. I spent six formative years growing up in Mexico and I've lived there twice as an adult. Time in Mexico is different; it's slower, as if moving in a long unhurried arc. In the United States, particularly in the north, it seems there is rarely enough time. There is a sense of people starving for time —in a rush, too much to do, drawn thin, overwhelmed, tense. Like being at a high altitude, people are gasping for time. In a land prosperous with belongings and stimulation, we are paupers when it comes to time.

I often start my classes by saying, "There is no rush, there is nowhere to get to, there is nothing that has to be done. Today, we have plenty of time." This is frequently followed by sighs and shoulders dropping a centimeter or two. We tend to brace against time, trying to pack so much into it that simply hearing that there is enough for the time being lets us begin to relax.

I used to complain in class that I wished I had more time. Then I realized that I was falling victim to wanting too much. Now my mantra is: do less. Whether I have a seven-hour workshop or a fifty-minute class, I have plenty of time. I often take down the clocks in the dance studio so that we can get out of clock time and enter body time.

I n The Time of Your Life workshop, I began by asking everyone how they relate to the idea that we have seven hours together. Do you see this time span as a straight line or a curved line? How does it feel to you? Do you picture time? Or feel it kinesthetically? Does time have texture for you? Is it like velvet, a water slide, itchy weeds, or is it rough like sandpaper?

We then did an awareness exercise that is effective for quieting the mind and becoming present. We wrap one hand around the thumb of the other hand. Letting the hands rest in the lap, we feel for the pulse in the thumb. When we find the pulse, we count backwards from ten to one on the beats of the pulse, and then feel a few more beats. We then change to the other thumb. Going back and forth we do every finger down to the pinkies.

I have found that this simple awareness of an interior rhythm allows something at the core to settle and the mind to become quieter. It's also a wonderful way to get to sleep at night when the mind-grinches want to keep you awake.

Most people "see" time as moving in a direction. In front of us is the future; behind us is the past. We hear phrases like "That is behind us now" and "We will see what lies ahead." I feel that this commonly held "view" of time has an effect on our dancing. It makes our movement more linear and symmetrical and less spherical and multifaceted.

I suggested to the class the image that time comes at us from every direction, from the entire sphere all at once, and disappears into the past inside us. Time surrounds us—we are consumers of time; we ingest it.

We used this image of time coming from every direction as a way to meditate on the threshold inside us, where time crosses over from the future, from the outside, to the past, on the inside. We "sit" in the cusp of time. This slight change in our view of time from linear to spherical had the effect of changing our perception of time from visual to kinesthetic. As we meditated on the passing of time, we played with putting the threshold where time passes into the past in the brain, in the heart, in the belly, in the groin, and at the skin. We made ourselves porous to time, feeling it as it passed into us.

From this place of awareness, of feeling time in motion, we began to move our bodies. We let the velocity of time move us. We filled our sails with time, looking for the pace where the movement was effortless.

When a person shouts into a canyon, each gorge has its own pitch at which an echo comes back the clearest. In the same way, each person has a rhythm in which they can move with lucidity and clarity. They do not *will* their movement along but rather *allow* velocity to move them. People can move for a long time once they find that rhythm. So, for a half hour, an hour, in the class, we moved, riding the brim of time.

This work evolved into partnering. With the complexities of a relationship that arises from working with a partner—expectations and judgments and reactions—it became difficult to keep our awareness on the passage of time. At first, we had to slow down. It took practice to quiet down enough internally to achieve a state where we could kinesthetically experience the dance with our partner as the embodiment of time passing.

At this point, the workshop turned a corner and the focus became how to stay in that quiet internal place while dancing in a variety of dynamics.

The Art of Waiting

I said to my soul, be still, and wait without hope
for hope would be hope for the wrong thing;

Wait without love
for love would be love of the wrong thing;

There is yet faith
but the faith and the love and the hope
are all in the waiting.

Wait without thought,
for you are not ready for thought:

So the darkness shall be the light,
and in the stillness the dancing.

—T. S. Eliot

Working with time led us down an unexpected back road into the act of waiting. I have experienced that the people who bring the broadest palette of colors to the dance bring a quiet thread at the core of their movement, a stillness. There is a sense that amidst the velocity and action, amidst the hurricane of activity, there is a quiet eye. I get the sense that there is a place in these dancers that is in the act of waiting.

The dictionary definition of "waiting" reads, in part: "*To be available or in readiness, to look forward eagerly, to stay or rest in expectation, to attend upon or escort, esp. as a sign of respect, to soar over ground until prey appears. Etymology: Old high German* wachton: *to be wide awake.*"

I relate to waiting as being "wide awake" and "in readiness." The idea of "soar[ing] over ground until prey appears" also pleases my imagination. The act of waiting is the act of soaring, in readiness, eyes wide open.

I've been looking for that quiet thread at the core for a long time. What seems like lifetimes ago, when I was in my early twenties, I lived for years at Zen Centers and spent time visiting monasteries in the Far East. This included a daily meditation practice and monthly retreats. What I found was that my mind loves to move and is not fond of sitting still.

When I discovered Contact Improvisation, it felt like I had walked into a house and knew where the furniture was—I felt like I was home. I resigned as director of the Empty Gate Zen Center in Berkeley, gave up my robes and bowls, and committed to a life of dancing. My constitution found it easier to become quiet while in motion than while trying to keep still with my butt propped up on a cushion.

When I left the Zen Center, I wanted to continue a regular practice. Knowing that movement was easier for me, I decided to do yoga. But I found a resistance to the long routine and could never keep it up. After a decade of off-again/on-again practice, I asked myself, why am I beating myself up about this? How can I find the pathway of ease? I played with different formats until I found that I could do six minutes of yoga each morning.

Six minutes. It works. I do it joyously. It feels like I could still do more, and the next day I'm happy to return. And over the decades, those six minutes kept doubling. By the time I'm 80 I expect to have a two-hour joyful practice daily.

From this research into what works to make a busy mind like

mine quieter, I've found other methods like the finger meditation described earlier. Most of these simple meditations ground a person somewhere in the body and the senses:

- listening to the farthest sound / listening to the sound right in the ears
- breathing through the mouth and nose simultaneously
- a slow soft self-caress
- the "small dance" of standing
- awareness of both the transition between the exhale and the inhale, and the transition between the inhale and the exhale

Another one of my favorites I learned from the Vipassana meditation teacher, Jack Kornfield—the raisin meditation. Take a raisin and keep it in your hand. Feel the weight of it. With a finger, feel the texture and density of the skin and pulp. Put it to your nose and become aware of the topography of the raisin's scent. Look into the valleys and peaks, the highlights and dark crevasses. Then put it in your mouth, close your eyes, and take a couple of minutes to get the full experience of eating a single raisin. Notice the trajectory of the flavor as it bursts forth, the flood of saliva, and the way the body's chemistry changes the flavor. Notice the aftertaste and the echoes of the aftertaste.

Doing this awareness exercise as a class warm-up opens up the body and faculties for C.I. As the senses awaken and open, the joints lubricate, creating a willingness to stay engaged in sensation as we go into movement.

We started the second afternoon of the workshop with the raisins. Continuing the awareness into the aftertaste is important in what it teaches us about waiting. When I dance with

someone who has the lucid quality of waiting, I notice that while
in motion they tend to broadcast where they have just been. They
are still tasting or hearing the echo of what was. As their dance
partner, I get the opportunity to relate to a range of possibilities—
where the movement appears to be going, where it is in the
moment, or where it just was.

To paint a picture of this: Imagine that you are dancing with a
partner and you are both on your feet and in physical contact.
Your partner begins to fold to the floor, softly creasing at the
ankles, knees, and pelvis. But as your partner folds down, he
leaves a hand up at your chest level. At this point, he might
continue to the floor or, by centering in the hand left behind,
spiral back up to standing. As his partner, you have a choice of
relating to the destination of the floor, to the dropping motion
itself, or to the hand that has stayed up in the air at your chest. By
leaving something behind, his movement opens up your choices
as well as his own. In each moment, there is a sense of relaxation
in the myriad of choices. And in that profusion of options, in that
generosity of possibilities, the cusp of the present gets wider. The
moment becomes more alive in all that it is offering.

When myriad possibilities appear in each moment, the opportunities for self-criticism go down. You are less likely to think, "Oh, I
missed that one," because there are many more than "one" to
choose from. The pathway you end up taking is simply what you
are contributing to the dance, and you're less caught up in ideas
of right and wrong.

For years I have wondered how I, how a person, can increase
their capacity to stay in this quiet core. What I increasingly
find is the need to let go of willful control, to drop the reins, to let
the animal brain and body have a stronger voice. There is an
inner dictator that demands resolution, a resolution that is fixed

and unchanging. He wants a single picture of the river rather than letting the river flow. (My inner dictator also wants the classes I teach to be entertaining.) How do we increase our capacity to live in the unresolved?

James Hillman talks about this state when he writes:

 But reaping these rewards requires learning to accept a self that remains ambiguous no matter how closely it is scrutinized. Fluid, active, filled with unresolvable contradictions, it is the nature of the self to remain beyond the ego's willful demand for a logically consistent system.

It's like hitchhiking by the side of the road. You don't know if you are going to get a ride in the next minute or in the next three days. It's throwing yourself into your destiny—part is choice and part is surrender.

In the second weekend of the workshop, we danced with the idea of leaving something behind by working with the idea of follow-through—letting each movement, each moment of the dance be the seed of the next. We attempted to calm our conscious and unconscious willfulness by allowing each instant to follow through rather than throwing in new impulses.

We also did exercises to build our capacity for staying in disorientation by continuing to follow through rather than re-center—even when we were off balance, up high, or in a moment of exhilaration. Especially in these moments, we tried to leave something behind, stay quiet at the core, continue with a sense of soaring over the ground, looking for prey—waiting.

During these two weekends, did time slow down? Had our

focused attention given us more day? The spherical quality of our time did make the present junctures seem wider, like there was more choice, more experience packed into each moment. But at the end of each day, we were all surprised that our time was up so soon.

2

THE EARTH IS BREATHING YOU

WHY WE PRACTICE TO CENTER AND GROUND

Imagine gazing up at a 30-floor building that is under construction. The structure towers 300 feet over you and is nothing but girders and steel beams. You take the freight elevator to the top floor and the doors slide open. Between you and your destination juts a 10-foot-long steel girder and a mild breeze. You look below through 300 feet of open space to the ground. People look like slow moving ants.

What do you do to prepare yourself to walk out on that beam? What do you do physically and emotionally to take the first step? How do you find a connection, even from way up here, to the ground?

This preparation is called centering and grounding. It's about coming home to yourself and your relationship with the constant influence of gravity. These skills are an essential step for developing responsiveness as a dancer. Until we know that firmness in our own two feet, it's difficult to feel confident in the rich world of being off balance and the unpredictability of shared centers with others.

Training for this moment is found in many disciplines. Some practices imagine the body's center about 2-3 inches below the navel, in the abdomen. If you dissect a body you won't find a gland or bone or star sapphire to mark the spot. But in relationship to the ground, the entire pelvic girdle can become a source of strength and connection that supports our movement.

A strong center can hold its ground. It is stable, rooted, can take a position of responsibility, face life squarely, be firm in its footing. It is content, without the need to go out and find justification for itself. It can wear robes and jewels and the crown of royalty – it can say, "Here I am!"

Learning to center and ground comes from a frequent returning to the core. One has to return under varying circumstances to become familiar with this place. In dance class, we start with controlled situations – then work with staying centered in more uncontrolled and chaotic conditions.

Imagery is an effective tool for this practice. We imagine attaching our pelvic girdle to the ground with a tap root, connecting to the middle of the turning earth, or to an artesian spring streaming up through our core. We might see ourselves as a granite mountain with crags and ledges, or we might stand and feel the earth is breathing us. As we sense the tug of gravity on our bodies it's helpful to imagine that at the same time gravity is pulling us from below, it is also pushing us from above. This puts us kinesthetically in the center, giving us a sense of being supported and held between two forces rather than one.

A common structure Contact Improvisation teachers use is the feather/boulder exercise. Half the class chooses to imagine that they are a feather or a boulder. The other half walks around and tries to pick these people up. As a boulder, the image leads a person to drop their center and move it away from their partner, making them heavier. As a feather, the person raises their center and puts it close to their partner's core, which makes them lighter. Each teaches us something about the other and both teach us the power of imagery.

After working with images and exercises for centering and grounding I like to test our abilities in increasingly challenging situations. One of my favorites, not only for what it teaches us about the power that comes from our centers, but also for the energy it generates in class, is the Two Against One exercise.

Two people stand tightly side by side. They cross their arms firmly against their rib cages. A third person, also with their arms crossed, pushes against the fronts of the duo. The job of the duo is to slowly push the single person backwards so the single person can feel the edge of their strength. The job of the single person is to attempt to push the two people backwards. The lesson is about finding ground and center and pushing with all the strength one can muster. Grunting and yelling are encouraged. (The word "grunt" comes from the same root as the words "ground" and "groin.")

Once this has been tried I show how imagination affects our abilities. I add a fourth person who stands behind the duo and holds a doll swaddled in a towel. I tell the single pusher that this fourth person is stealing his baby. And not only that, but he has a fire-filled pit behind him. It's amazing to see what these images do to a person's ability to find strength. I've sometimes seen the duo end up flattened against the wall.

In another exercise called Push and Drop, one person stands with their feet shoulder-distance apart and imagines sending down roots. The second person, the assistant, introduces her hand to some part of the standing body and begins to push. The receiver meets the push with an equal amount of force to stay centered. The assistant pushes on the torso, the limbs and the head as the receiver attempts to track the pathway up through their body from the ground to the pushing hand.

Then the rules change. The pusher, without warning, pulls her hand away. The receiver, to not fall into the hole created by the sudden absence of the pushing, needs to reverse the pathway in the body to the ground.

Normally, when we lose our balance we fling our arms up in the air and rise to regain our center. This exercise teaches us to drop back down along our connection to the ground. It teaches us that the pathway that came up to meet an outside force can, with awareness, be the same pathway that brings us back to balance.

To continue the practice of this, sometimes I will take the class out to railroad tracks to walk the rails. This is one of the most basic meditations, done by many of us as adolescents, for learning to drop our center and come into ourselves.

Polycentric Dancing

Why do we learn to center and ground? To improvise. To have the basis to take risks, to enter (center in) the unknown, to build our capacity for the unresolved so that we can spontaneously, extemporaneously, creatively unfold and improvise in the present.

One dilemma with teaching exercises for centering and grounding is that they can make people rigid in their dancing. I give the caveat that this is only a stepping stone to build trust in ourselves for more dynamic situations. We want to develop a relationship with gravity that assists us at all times including when off-balance and during flight. And we want that connection to stay alive and sensitive when we start working with a partner and share a mutual non-proprietary relationship to the earth we dance on.

When people learn Contact Improvisation I delight as their dance evolves from "centered" to "polycentric." I begin to see their limbs and torso and head moving autonomously. They pitch off-center without knowing how the motion will resolve itself. They enter spirals that extend past the body, and different body parts fall *and* rise simultaneously. They have begun to bravely improvise.

This is the transition where they begin to take their grounding less preciously. Where they become strong enough in their own self to know when to stand firm, when to bend and when to blow away like tumbleweed. They begin to ground not only in themselves, but in fear, in excitement, in imagination, in paradox.

Over the years, when I have taught a workshop focused on a single theme, I've frequently been amazed at the detours and side trips we get taken on. I begin a workshop on the theme of weight exchange, and find that I'm actually gaining entry into the worlds of momentum, entropy and centrifugal force; not to mention the sub-worlds of arches, apexes, arcs, and under-arcs. And I had thought we were just going to work with the skill of passing weight through the bones.

The same has been true when I've focused on the theme of centering and grounding. The act of moving to center, finding a relationship to the ground, often leads into its opposites – being off-center and in states of disorientation.

When we are beginners at Contact Improvisation we tend to dance with our feet planted in a wide base in anticipation of supporting someone's mass. The wide base creates stability that can bear weight. But I've noticed that as a person matures in their dancing their base narrows. When we stand with our feet close together we can respond more quickly to the invitations that come during the dance, including moving to a wide base when necessary. The feet become like a school of fish, able to move any which way on the floor. The dancer becomes light in their step, nomadic, adaptable, ready to fly as soon as they land.

In order to organize ourselves with another person's weight we start with the idea that we need to brace ourselves. It's crucial to know we have this ability. As a person develops their dancing skills they learn that a partner's mass is taken more easily on the move. As soon as we take a solid position we deny ourselves the help the arriving weight is offering us. By moving the weight into our center and moving with it, we are much more in control and use less exertion along the way.

If you pick up a kitchen chair and hold it at arm's reach, it is going to feel heavier than if you hug it to your belly. If someone tosses a chair to you, it is easier to catch it by blending with its trajectory rather than putting your arms out and stopping it cold. To join the trajectory of the chair it helps if the body is already in a state of readiness and mobility. We are closer to this state from a narrow base. We are more able to deal with large masses of moving weight from a fluid, multi-centered place than a "grounded" place.

To give students a physical example of multiple centers I take the Push and Drop exercise another step. When the hand that has been pushing suddenly disappears, rather than reversing the pathway to the ground, we let that center fall into the hole. Meanwhile, another center can take over from its relationship to the ground to bring us to balance. If someone is pushing on the front of your shoulder and that hand suddenly disappears, that shoulder can follow into the hole that's created. At the same time your other shoulder or a hip goes backwards counterbalancing the forward motion. In this exercise, the body fills with spirals and we can act and react from many centers along or within these spirals.

To help this polycentric dance I embellish the image of gravity pushing from above as well as pulling from below. I further imagine that gravity comes from every direction. It's a sphere of force. It's what holds my skin on. Now I can relate to all directions and not just my verticality. A sense of spherical gravity gives the support that helps to keep me organized when I'm off-balance.

When my dance partner and I move through the room and I sense he's on a trajectory that invites me to become airborne, and suddenly that invitation has me flying upside down with my head below my pelvis, my adrenals at full throttle, I need to remember that when I arrive at the apex, he may not be there to catch me. In these moments, I imagine myself being caught by space itself. By making space tangible the arc of time slows down. The extra time allows me to relate different centers to the ground, to make contact with my partner's movement, to choose between the possibilities of rolling, sloughing, flipping or whatever else presents itself in the moment. This spherical sense of gravity and space is a small image that makes a big difference.

To center and ground simultaneously in more than one center takes the courage to live in the tension created by paradox. It's the feeling that the dance is askew. It's being in an impeccable room and not straightening the crooked picture. When we have multiple views of what we engage in, multiple pathways open up. Now we are centering not only in the physical, but also in our relationship with our partner, in the emotional body, and in the imagination. And they sometimes disagree.

Polycentricity is not about making things complicated. It's also not about coercing things to be simple.

It is through grounding that the tension of maintaining multiple centers becomes tolerable. We give up a solitary relationship to the ground, to our partner, to our self-image. The rapport *or* non-rapport of each center allows for an association between the different and sometimes competing focal points.

In this state of multiplicity, the improvisation moves from being purely about physics into the rich and fluid realms of relationships.

Once again, an image is helpful here. Imagine that there are many little people that live in your chest. Some are skilled at coming out and being the center of attention. Some are superb at dancing on tables and singing in front of the party. There are others who live in your chest who have no legs. Some have gnarled and disfigured faces. Some would rather die than be seen.

There's a whole menagerie living and breathing in there.

The idea of being centered and grounded can be an assault on these little people – the little hard-to-hear voices in our lives. Inside we are many; the one who leads, the one who follows, the one who grieves, the one who's always strong.... These little ones don't always agree and when added up, we are not big enough to contain them all. Allowing the little ones their full place calls for a bigger view of ourselves. We are a pantheon of possibilities, but when we ground in a single center we slice off the intelligence and expressions of these little chest dwellers, what D.H. Lawrence refers to when he says:

> Oh when man has escaped from the barbed-wire
> entanglement

of his own ideas and his own mechanical devices
there is a marvelous rich world of contact and sheer
*   fluid beauty*
and fearless face-to-face awareness of now-naked life
and me, and you, and other men and women
and grapes, and ghouls, and ghosts and green
*   moonlight*
and ruddy-orange limbs stirring the limbo
of the unknown air, and eyes so soft
softer than the space between the stars,
and all things, and nothing, and being and not-being
alternately palpitant

When we encounter others who have little people in their chest that find a way to get in and meet our little people, and we get to visit their hidden ones, then we have made contact, then there is chemistry.

By letting ourselves have many centers, many voices, many colors, we find ourselves in a multi-layered, richly woven tapestry of improvisation. It's here that we begin to meet over the breadth and depths of who we are. And while centering and grounding are useful skills to build self-trust, they can feed into our willfulness. That willfulness, both conscious and unconscious, is part of the colonization that doesn't allow the little ones to nourish the improvisation. Seasoned improvisers dance with their little people. By dropping the reins, by entering the dance with a polycentric willingness, worlds and connections open up that we could not have intended or imagined.

(Thanks to Malcolm Manning for giving me the image: the earth is breathing you.)

3

101 WAYS TO SAY NO TO CONTACT IMPROVISATION

BOUNDARIES AND TRUST

... it is important that awake people be awake,
or a breaking line may discourage them back to sleep;
the signals we give–yes or no, or maybe–
should be clear: the darkness around us is deep.

William Stafford

Contact Improvisation is a dance that invites our entire body and being to be present and available. To dance this form, we need to build a capacity for trust with ourselves and our partners. We nurture or harm that trust by our ability or inability to set and respect boundaries.

This process is ongoing for me even after four decades of dancing. At different points along the way, I've grappled with many questions: How do you let people know you are not warmed up and not yet ready to dance, or that you want to end a dance? How do you set boundaries when you have a physical limitation or are

working with an injury, or are dancing with an insensitive partner? What do you do when your lover is having a sensual dance
with someone else and you are feeling vulnerable? How do you
intercede when a group of musicians are all looking at each other
and having a fabulous time, but have forgotten the dancers they
are playing for? How do you communicate to a duet that their
loud, emotional catharsis is overpowering and interfering with
the other dances in the room? How are these boundaries negoti-
ated and communicated?

A student came into a workshop of mine with a flaming rash all
over his body. When I said, "Find a partner," everyone fled from
where he was standing, so I ended up working with him. I was
uncomfortable that his rash might be infectious, so I asked him
directly, "Is this contagious?" He said he had an allergic reaction
called mastocytosis that releases massive amounts of histamines,
which cause the skin discoloration. He spoke of his long struggle
with it and said it was definitely not transmittable. I was relieved,
and as I had hoped, the class eavesdropped and he had little
trouble finding partners after that.

A friend and dance partner came to the Philadelphia Contact
Festival where I was teaching and performing. We were looking
forward to dancing together, and at the closing jam we finally had
our chance. As we danced, different people approached us to join
in. A couple of times we were able to communicate physically
that we were not done yet. When one person tried to join I said,
"We have had a date for this duet for six weeks and we still need
some more time together." I checked in with that person later and
she said my "no" was communicated clearly and gracefully.

I've found instances in which the community comes together
to help individuals set boundaries. In the mid-1980s, many
women who danced at the weekly Contact jam in Berkeley, Cali-

fornia, complained about a particular man who regularly came to dance. I will call him Roland. They said dancing with him was unpleasant because of his lack of awareness of boundaries. It was difficult for the women to describe the behavior they didn't like; they could only call it a "feeling".

One said, "Dancing with Roland is like dancing with an overly enthusiastic puppy, the one that's trying to hump your shins." The general feeling was that he was "getting off" on the dance, and stealing something that was not being offered by his partners.

It was not hard to notice that almost every time a young woman came through the door of the jam for the first time, from wherever he was in the room, Roland's head would pop up. Within minutes he would be at her side, offering to enlighten her on the finer points of Contact Improvisation. Many of those women were never seen at the jam again.

Though many women could talk about Roland, it turned out that most had not said anything directly to him. It was confusing for them to get this cloying feeling from this man and yet have so little specific behavior to talk to him about. I remember one woman saying, "Talking to him would be like complaining about the weather; it wouldn't do any good."

Roland would regularly attend the Northern California Contact Jam, a five-day residential jam at Harbin Hot Springs. Here I learned a lesson about communicating boundaries from one of the organizers, Sue Stuart. One evening I was present as two women sat down with Sue to lament about Roland. They wanted her to do something about him.

Sue asked, "Have you said anything to Roland directly?" When she heard that they hadn't, she asked, "What would you like to say to him?" Both articulated what they would say. One said, "I feel you are getting off sexually while dancing with me, and I don't want to dance with you or be approached by you until you get your sexual desires under control." From saying it aloud, the woman was able to take Roland aside and talk to him. The other didn't want to confront him directly until Sue offered to accompany her and be at her side.

I was impressed that Sue responded to these women by giving them the means to take care of the predicament themselves rather than letting them give their power to her, the person in the position of authority. Roland apologized and said he would change his behavior.

A few months later it was clear that Roland had changed his dancing with the women who were regulars in the community. Yet his radar would still light up when new women came into the weekly jam. The seasoned women dancers in the community began to take responsibility to dance with the newcomers before Roland got to them.

A few of the men, including myself, took Roland aside and with good humor told him what we perceived. We said he was harming the community and needed to stop this conduct or stop coming to the jams. While we approached him with some levity, he understood the gravity of the situation by the fact that so many of us had made the same observation and were speaking of the same consequences. Roland did change and now, over three decades later, still regularly dances in a welcoming community.

In this instance, it worked out well for both Roland and the group. However, I've heard of similar situations with both men and women that weren't so successful; the individuals involved were finally asked not to return.

There are also the Contact teachers who troll. A friend was

hosting one of these well-known teachers to lead a workshop in the Boulder community. I asked her, "Are you aware of this teacher's history?" She responded, "We told him we are aware of his behavior and gave him the condition that he not get sexual with any student during the workshop, OR groom the students for afterwards. He accepted these conditions." It was brave and necessary for her to be this clear.

Sexuality is messy and will always be a perennial issue in our dance community. It is not unusual for a local jam to go through a reckoning around boundaries being transgressed. Some jams now have jam rule documents and release forms as a result of these reckonings.

Having the strength and wisdom to address issues before they escalate is the preferred option. The seasoned women taking responsibility to track and dance with female newcomers and the seasoned men taking responsibility to keep an eye out for the men's conduct are helpful steps. Neige Christenson and Max Gautier of the Boston community joke that they at times need to go into "vigil-auntie" mode. Earthdance has made efforts to make a network of "resource" people available to jammers. They are chosen from the staff at Earthdance and also from the attendees who are therapists or others deemed reliable, approachable people with whom attendees can talk about issue that arise, from boundary crossing to loneliness.

From my ongoing inquiry into what's needed to cultivate clear boundaries, I've developed a workshop called "101 Ways to Say No to Contact Improvisation." The premise of the workshop is that until a person has the confidence and ability to say no to something, they won't have the trust and capacity to fully say yes to it. In the workshop, we explore physical and verbal skills to say no to dances, to touch, to being lifted, to weight exchange, to momentum, and to manipulation.

For example, when someone reaches to grab me and lift me up and I don't want to be lifted, I can drop my weight and move my center away from my partner's center. I become too heavy to lift. I have clearly said no. With this knowledge of how to say no, I can extrapolate the opposite; when I want to say yes and take the opportunity to fly up, I already have the sense of how to become light by raising my center and organizing it over my partner's core.

The same is true with touch. I need the self-trust and ability to remove someone's hand (either physically or verbally) when I don't want their physical contact or manipulation. With confidence in my ability to set the boundary, I can choose the opposite and open up to the touch.

Robert Bly offers us an image in *A Little Book on the Human Shadow*. It is that we have a door in our psyche. As children, the doorknob is on the outside and people come and go as they please. The adults feed us, they wipe our butts, they carry us around. As we mature into adults, we learn to transfer the doorknob to the inside and choose when and for whom to open and close the door. If we know we can close the door, we are freer to open it and invite people in.

Some people come to this dance form and it's a challenge for them to feel and connect to the sensations in their body. This can be a result of people having forced their way through their door early on in life. For those whose boundaries were splintered as children, it can be as if they've created a shield or protective armor that keeps them from making full contact with their bodies and with the world. Here it becomes important for them to develop boundary-setting skills, to know they have the doorknob on the inside. With the ability to express limits, they can begin to relinquish the protective layers and invite more possibilities into the Contact dance and, furthermore, into their lives.

Contact Improvisation has a basic principle that each person takes responsibility for themselves. I am the only person who can be inside my body, so I need to keep a part of me awake – the part that can sense and communicate (physically or verbally) my needs, limits, and desires. I need to keep myself safe and from here I can begin to care for the group. Adhering to a practice of this principle is one way to move the doorknob to the inside.

During the 101 Ways to Say No workshop, I teach another safety skill; this one for learning to communicate quickly in high-energy situations. We learn to shout one-syllable words that demand immediate attention: "Stop!" "Back!" "Wait!" (I don't use "No!" anymore because it's a word rich in nuance and, as anybody with children knows, a word prone to be tested.) We also practice exclaiming words that specify a part of the body that is in pain or about to be: "Knee!" "Ankle!" "Neck!" It's rare that this skill will be used, but knowing that the words are in place reassures the psyche and allows us to open the door to more athletic, acrobatic, and disorienting dances.

As I developed material for the workshop, I wanted an exercise that would clearly demonstrate that a person's ability to say no would create a greater capacity for yes. Out of this investigation came an exercise called "Two Rivers."

I don't introduce this exercise until the group has some history of working together. One person, the receiver, lies on their back. Two others, the "two rivers," give the receiver slow flowing caresses directed by arm signals from the receiver. When the receiver crosses their arms over their torso, it means "Don't touch me at all." When they rest their arms on the floor beside their body, it means "Touch me nicely, like you would if we were in a public place." When they place their arms on the floor over their head, it means "You can touch me anywhere and everywhere, no-holds-barred." The receiver can change the position of their arms at any time.

The touch might have a calming tone, a nurturing tone, a sensual tone, or a sexual tone, but the receiver is always in control of what they are is receiving. The receiver opens and closes the locks on the rivers. The receiver is instructed that they have one rule: at some point they have to say no to the touch.

The two rivers are instructed that no matter where the receiver's arms are, they should only touch to their level of comfort. The two rivers also get to chaperone each other. In case one river doesn't notice the receiver has crossed their arms, the other river will let them know.

It is clear to participants that if this exercise didn't contain the full stop, "No, don't touch me anywhere," it wouldn't be able to offer the full yes to touch everywhere. With the boundary available and visible, people are able to ask for more than if the boundary wasn't in place. With all the implicit consensuality in our dance form, practicing an explicit consensuality allows for more comfort with the tacit agreements we make in each moment as we dance.

S teve Paxton has been known to say, "Contact Improvisation is not a gland game," meaning, in part, that it's not a sexual dance. I often hear people say, "I love this dance form because it's a non-sexual way to be physical and affectionate and playful with people."

This is not true for me. I am always aware of myself as a sexual being. Every breath I take is sexual. There is a rapture I feel when

I'm dancing with women and a pride I feel in being a man when I dance with men. I can't amputate that part of myself.

I certainly don't want my partners to feel I'm using the dance to "get off." Sometimes I dance with the image that my partner and I are in a one-hundred-year courtship. We are not trying to get anywhere. Without closing down any part of myself, I can dance with that savory side of me awake. Authentic, spontaneous contact entails surrendering the need to gain or profit from the exchange. In this surrender, a person can dance this form and keep their sexuality alive.

Whenever we dance, there is a testing of what is consensual. Will you accept my weight? Can we go fast? Can we go very, very slow? Occasionally I meet someone and we consensually bring an erotic or seductive energy to the dance. We move in concentrically and test what is welcome for both of us. There is a safety in the exchange because we are chaperoned by our sense of appropriate behavior in the jam environment.

When I'm in the backyard of our home watching our children play with friends, their improvised games are a constant setting and testing of boundaries. Sometimes in their play they are famous paleontologists digging up the biggest dinosaur ever discovered. Sometimes they are empire builders – running around with their swords and cardboard shields, crawling on their bellies into forts under the hedges – making and breaking and negotiating the rules as they go. Sometimes it's a physical cue or a single word; sometimes the play stops completely as they work out the rules of the game. They are continually working to make the flow of attention and power be fair and balanced. It looks similar to what we do in our dance community.

There has been an ongoing negotiation of boundaries over the years at the Northern California Contact Jam. The group wrangles over how much structure to have, how much emotional catharsis or music is desirable in the jam space. Over the course of the first ten or so jams, as we established our spoken and unspoken agreements, we had many instances of crossing into argument. We learned over time that listening to one another was what was needed to find a balance between opposing desires. There was little need for executive decisions. Being in the conflict and hearing each person speak allowed for solutions to evolve naturally.

I noticed that the jams with the most open disagreement also had the most sincere and tearful gratitude at the end. When we were fully involved in the testing and establishing of boundaries, there was a sense of learning, of creating relationships, of being in an alive group that left us with a profound sense of appreciation for one another.

Being in a group of dancers and doing this ongoing work of clarifying boundaries is like inhabiting a rock tumbler – those containers you fill with stones and spin for days so that the stones polish one another. As we learn to sense and express our boundaries, we tumble and rub and hit against others both physically and figuratively. It can hurt as our sharp edges get rounded, but over time we become polished, slowly revealing the precious gems we carry. Through this process we begin to treasure the living entity called "community" that helps us develop a greater capacity for yes – in our dance and in our lives.

4

MUSINGS ON BEING A TOURING CONTACT ARTIST

B erlin, Germany
July 15, 1999

On the road again. For five of the past eight months I've taught and performed Contact Improvisation in twelve cities, in six countries, on four continents. I'm road-fatigued. Recently, during moments of quiet recently I've been asking myself: What am I really doing as I tour? What's the appeal? What makes me want to stop? After decades of being engaged with this dance form, could I possibly be looking at another twenty years?

I'm sitting at a makeshift desk in the K77 Project, a squatter's tenement in East Berlin. After the Berlin wall came down, people from West Berlin flooded into the East to squat the empty buildings. Most were evicted immediately. But not the people who moved in here.

Freedom of expression and the arts are strongly protected under the German constitution. Knowing this, a group of squatters turned the takeover of this building into a performance piece. In every window of the three-story building, someone dressed as a doctor or nurse held a rope that led to a person on the street dressed as a giant heart. To the beat of drums, this motley medical crew performed a "heart transplant," infusing new life into the oldest building in the neighborhood. And because the group was exercising their right of artistic expression, they weren't arrested and weren't evicted. They did theater here on and off as they continued to negotiate with the government. Within three years, their occupancy was legalized.

If I didn't tour I wouldn't know this place existed or that this had ever happened.

The class I'm teaching is held in the back building in a dance studio that is part of the collective. I'm doing a five-day workshop at the invitation of Stephanie Maher, one of a handful dancers I know who has moved to Europe from the USA.

In four nights here so far, I've been moved into a different bedroom three times. Tonight I'm to sleep in a trailer in the backyard. I am feeling what has become a familiar sense of displacement.

For years I rarely toured. I observed the people who spent a lot of time on the road and saw the toll it took on their relationships. But I've been touring more in the past three years since I moved to San Miguel de Allende in Mexico. There's a lot of coming and going in my new home, and it's easy to flow into a more itinerant lifestyle. I've also needed the money.

One day a few years ago, I noticed an article in USA Today that ranked the ten best and the ten worst professions. The U.S. Department of Labor had chosen five criteria to judge people's occupations: growth potential of the profession, stress level, likelihood of injury, income potential and the possibility for advancement. Six of the top ten were in the computer field. In the bottom ten, in fact second from the worst occupation was - can you guess

- "dancer." None of the other arts even ranked in the bottom ten. According to the USDL, the only career worse than dancing is logging.

When I read that article, I had just come from a rehearsal and couldn't stop laughing. How could I have chosen this profession? I certainly understood why it showed up in the bottom 10, economically speaking. But where would dancing rank if one of the measures they'd used had been the intangible criterion of job satisfaction?

I imagine that the criterion of "likelihood of injury" was a major factor in the USDL putting dance in this position. Most of the professional Contacters I know do not have health insurance unless they come from a country where the government provides it for free. It's an expense I've shouldered, and when years ago I broke my arm on a badly rippled Marley dance floor, I was relieved I'd made that choice.

Oakland, California
July 30

It's comfortable here—I'm house-sitting in the familiar home of a close friend. Her two cats are in my lap; one is asleep and the other is looking at me oddly. I'm teaching a three-week C.I. training intensive in San Francisco with Ray Chung. We have participants from seven countries. Today Ray had us pay attention to the habitual ways we initiate physical contact during a dance. He then had us teach our particular styles to our partner. We then danced again, using our partner's ways of initiating. It was a good pattern-breaker.

Now both cats are looking at me. The tabby places his paw on my hand seeking equal time. I've been thinking about the rewards of touring. First, I get to see the world, not as a tourist but as someone who is personally invited into the cultures and subcultures of the places I visit. Generally, a group of people are gathered for a workshop, I'm flown in, driven around, fed the local cuisine, and given a bed. I have the privilege of teaching a form I cherish, and I am appreciated and paid for it. I get to meet wonderful and generous people and continue to develop my relationship with this dance.

On the other hand, after a while I lose a sense of place. What city am I in now? What bed? And some of those beds sag to the floor or are made of moldy thatched straw. Sometimes I've stayed with families where an imminent divorce poisons the atmosphere or the children are berated. Then there's the changing diet, the jet lag, phone adapters, cigarette smoke, the exhaustion from too many late nights, and encounters where the connection goes no further than chit-chat. And before any of that starts, there's the preparation for going on tour: packing, finding people to take care of my cat, manage the house, pay the bills... and then having to say goodbye again.

Then there are the business details, which can make even the most exhilarating tours difficult. A couple of times organizers have canceled a workshop at short notice because they weren't able to get enough participants or the funding they were planning on. Then the painful conversation has to happen about who is responsible for the airline ticket I'm holding and the time that was spoken for. Now I get the flight money sent to me in advance.

In one city, after finishing an under-enrolled workshop, I moved to a hotel because the home my host had found for me was filled with cockroaches. That day, they had also lost their resident boa constrictor in the room I was to sleep in. I was relieved to finally be by myself in the hotel, and I plugged in my computer to pick up my e-mail. Then poof!—my computer modem went up in a puff of smoke because they had a digital phone system. That was a bad tour day.

Boulder, Colorado
August 19

I'm sitting on the floor in a cabin perched up in the foothills of the Rocky Mountains. At night, I can sometimes hear the other-worldly wail of a puma. Down through the valley I can see the lights of Denver. Yesterday I finished a three-day workshop. It was supposed to run for five days, but not enough people signed up. As a way to entice more participants, the workshop was shortened. Today I have some unexpected time to write.

As I look over these musings, I see that most of the problems I have with being a touring Contact artist relate to the traveling and not the teaching and dancing. If the dance community were large enough in San Miguel, I would do most of my teaching at home and travel only on occasion. The low cost of living in Mexico allows me to live on a dancer's salary, but I still have to go abroad to get that income.

Even with the frustrations of traveling, I have enjoyed the interactions with the different people and seeing how they live. I'm getting a taste for the different styles of government and culture, for the ongoing effects of colonialism, and the newer impact of the spread of democracy. And through all my interactions with people, I've been surprised to find that touring gives me increasing hope for the future.

And I'm humbled by the generosity of people. Though I've occasionally had to suffer through some uncomfortable situations, mostly I've been fortunate to be welcomed by people who understand the archetype of being a host. It means a lot to take someone into your home. After I've been teaching all day, I find I need a room where I can close the door and be apart. I need some comfort, and I need time alone. I can no longer sleep on living-room floors with the dog that wants to go for a walk at 5 am. Most hosts understand this. How many times have they given me their bed and slept in the living room?

I think often about the people who are on the other side of the equation from me—the organizers. Gabriela Entin and Cristina Turdo, for example, who have brought several dance instructors to Buenos Aires, have talked to me about the different needs that different teachers have. One afternoon as we sat in the kitchen drinking yerba maté, they told me that some teachers arrive needing to know that their living situation is taken care of and need to get settled right away. Some have to see the studio. Some are concerned that the money is in order, and some need a great deal of acknowledgment. I asked them if I had been demanding. They laughed and said, "Less than some, more than others."

Acadia National Park, Maine
August 28

This is my third day walking trails and swimming in clear lakes overlooking the Atlantic Ocean. I'm not teaching here. I came to be with a good friend and to spend time in the wilderness. Another plus of touring is the opportunity to experience some of the world's natural wonders between engagements. It's in places like this that I get recharged.

I've been reflecting on what aspects of touring are the most fulfilling for me. I realize how much I love to see students increase their capacity for sensation and risk, to see them dancing less with their ideal and more with their partner. There is the satisfaction of watching someone who has learned to go

into flight without tensing their legs. And the profound gratification of introducing Contact to those few who realize they have
found the dance form they were seeking all their lives.

Last year I taught a master class in a high school for the
performing arts in the Midwest. While demonstrating with one
of the students, we got separated and my hand invited her into
the air. She flew feet first into the under-arc and weightlessly
landed on my hip. She did not plan—she allowed herself to fly.

The next day after class she told me that her mother was drug
addicted and mentally ill, her father in prison for child abuse.
She tearfully confided that in her life she had no one she could
trust except one friend who lives in a town 150 miles away. She
said that when we danced together, she'd trusted a new acquain-
tance for the first time in her life and that it had rocked her to the
core. Hearing her experience rocked me to the core, that this
dance form—and myself as one of its ambassadors—could have
such a profound effect on someone's life. It bears perhaps the
strongest testimony to why I keep teaching and performing.

San Miguel de Allende, Mexico
September 2

After two months on the road, I'm back home in Mexico. Once
again, I'm standing at my standing desk, where everything I need
is within arm's reach. Outside the bougainvillea vines are show-
ering the yard in purple, orange, and red. I can see the crooked
necks of the herons as they fly overhead on their way back to
their nests.

I just returned from what was supposed to be a thirteen-week
tour. Before I left, I rescheduled five of those weeks to next year

because of exhaustion. This move kept me from getting to where I would dislike going on tour and even the dance form itself.

Sometimes the hardest part of touring is returning home. After many glorious months on the road where my role in life is clear, it can be disorienting to return to San Miguel.

I do my usual routine to ground me: I go to Escondido Place to soak in the hot springs, I visit the botanical gardens to see the sunset over the desert, I settle in with a tub or two of chocolate ice cream.

But still, it's hard to recognize myself. When I travel from city to city, I know who I am: the touring Contact artist. I seem to know that one well. Then suddenly I'm back in my home and I can't identify so closely with that role. That's when the king dragon of questions again rears its head: Who am I?

When I'm in town I teach in Spanish at the National School of Fine Arts. My teaching style is imagistic rather than anatomical. It's rare to hear me talk about the psoas or proprioceptors, but you will hear me refer to the string of pearls that runs down the spine or the soap bubbles that make the joints slippery inside. When I'm teaching in English and I give an image, I can see the tremor of recognition go through about half the class. But because Spanish is a more metaphorical language, when I speak an image in Spanish I can see the tremor run through almost everybody.

My teaching is more experimental when I teach at home—I take some wild detours to see where they go. When I'm on tour, I'm more likely to do my "tried and true." Funny...when I first wrote that, I put down "tired and true." Mmmm.

El Charco del Ingenio, Botanical Gardens
Outside San Miguel de Allende

September 5

I'm sitting on my favorite boulder overlooking a canyon with vertical cliffs that fall into pools of water surrounded by clusters of mesquite trees. In winter, thousands of white-throated swifts arrive every night at sunset. They fill the sky and swirl above the canyon until they take a sudden dive in perfect formation spiraling into caves with openings about a hand's width across. After a few minutes, there is not a bird in the sky. This is a good place to get quiet.

Contact Improvisation is difficult to describe. We keep printing definitions in Contact Quarterly magazine because no single definition can contain this dance. It's like fire—always changing, and always manifesting in different forms. There's candlelight by the bedside, and crackling bonfires on the beach; there are forest fires that rage for miles, and the small hearth that warms the room. It's continually changing, and it's the same with C.I. And it has its own life cycle, from the warm-up to the listening and tracking, to the wild adrenaline dancing, to the cool-down. And not always in that order. I love this form, and I love seeing people inspired by the mystery of this dance.

But there's another, more hidden side to my relationship with C.I. I'm not sure I'm capable of or willing to do anything else. I'm somehow constitutionally fit for this kind of dancing. I'm not good at repetition, and finding this dance form that has no steps, an improvised dance where I can at least imagine that it's always new... well, it's like fire. And I'm happy here, in the midst of it.

But sometimes I just want to yell at C.I., "Damn you! Why aren't you more restrained, more predictable, so that I can understand you and move on? But no, you remain wild and mysterious and I need to keep digging to see what more is possible—in you and in me." Of course, if it were a tidy dance form with neat little phrases and counts, I probably never would have gotten involved with it in the first place.

I've heard that farmers who plant domesticated wheat have a vitally important task to do every few years if they want their crops to flourish. They must go into the wilderness and find wild wheat to take back to their farm and mix with their cultivated strain. The wild wheat gives the domesticated wheat more genetic diversity, which gives it endurance, strength, and a pleasing taste. I'm beginning to think of touring Contact artists as the wild wheat. We go into a community and introduce a wild strain into what has been locally cultivated.

But the opposite is also true. The act of going from place to place and dancing with different people impregnates my dancing with a quality that would be missing if I stayed at home.

I have four months here before my next tour. In the long run, will I continue this way of life? I don't know. It's rich, and it's hard. At the moment, I can't imagine what could be more satisfying or tiring. For now, I'm keeping the questions and inquiry alive. The mystery and the wildness at the center of Contact Improvisation are so close to my own center, that it's hard to imagine being able to resist.

5

JALAPEÑO PEPPERS IN THE BLOOD

DANCING WITH IMAGERY

Careful all ye who enter here. This essay is a web of metaphors, a fecund pond of water striders and leaf mush, bottom slime and the sudden undulating tail of a pollywog vanishing into the dark. I breathe images, they are the ether I live in, the substance I inhale and exhale. They are a vital and essential part of this man's dancing, teaching, and life.

How can images give succor to our dancing? When students trudge into class on Thursday evening tired from their day and their week they might assume that finding any vitality would be hopeless.

We begin class by imagining slippery soap bubbles multiplying in the joints, the ankles, knees, the pelvis. Glossy, reflective soap bubbles appear between each vertebra. Slick bubbles in between the ribs and under the shoulder blades. These bubbles make it easier and more pleasurable to be in motion than to be in stillness. The room becomes a swelling swirl of moving bodies.

Where before there was little access, the images now make a bridge into sensation. Yet we don't stop there. When the students realize that as they concocted their soapy, slippery mixture they grabbed the wrong bottle and added tequila to the soap, the joints become intoxicated (even though each person stays lucid and sober at the core and safely knows where everybody is in the room.) Unexpectedly, the body is socially lubricated, perhaps moving like it never has moved before...

And at this point we have barely begun the warm-up.

There are times we might feel lethargic or immobilized by our life's circumstances. Our emotional body might be at loggerheads with our desire to dance. Images can create bridges to other parts of ourselves where there are hidden resources. We find ourselves at the well, or better yet the artesian hot springs. And where we thought there was little possibility of movement or engagement, once we have soaked our tired muscles and swum under the waterfall, we find that we are ready to engage and sweat and play.

Images do not work for everybody. Some people have no doorway in their psyche for images; their skin is porous to other input but not imagery. But for those who are rocked by imagery, they work in the same way as memorized poems – it is like a time-release vitamin that continues nourishing you as long as you have it inside you. If you can find the images that feed you where you are deficient, be it vitamin D, or iodine, or compassion, or alertness, the results can be especially startling. Images can awaken parts of our personality that we didn't have access to before. They can shine a light on some part of us that we typically can't see. The right image can penetrate a person to the core.

Dance teachers use different lenses and styles of language when they teach. Some use an anatomical vocabulary. Some see the dance through the lens of the psychology of relationship. There are teachers whose vocabulary is kinesthetic and teachers who give a series of specific tasks. There are those who use the language of play and teach with a series of games. I tell my students that they ought to work with as many teachers as possible. This way they will find those who speak a language they can understand and learn from.

My portal into the body is not through anatomy books. Often Contact teachers talk about the flow of synovial fluid and the relationship of the atlas to the axis at the base of the skull. While I learn a great deal in their classes, my attempts to use this language have been like having a bone stuck in my throat. Rather than talk about vertebrae I'm far more likely to talk about the string of pearls that is the spine. Rather than referring to the discs of the spinal column, I'm more likely to ask people to notice the slimy oysters or melting pads of butter between those pearls.

In my classes I create an imagistic world, a narrative in which all of our sensing and investigation and activity exist. That world gets set up during the warmup and continues to be the cornerstone for the material through the rest of class.

I work with images in my own dancing. For years while improvising I would invoke the image of the cloak of invisibility, which allowed me to dance lightly despite my almost 200 pounds.

After both my parents and a best friend died within a short period, it was difficult for me to go and dance at jams. Sensing my body while dancing often led to weeping. But this image appeared: bones softened by grief. This gave me a tool that allowed me to not abandon my current feeling state but have it support the dancing.

When I find I'm laboring in the dance I invoke the image that I'm riding a bicycle downhill. I don't even have to peddle and I've got the wind on my face. I enjoy the image that my body is a jungle. The contact point fills with a rich diversity of wildlife and terrains that have yet to be discovered.

For a couple of years I invoked this image: sleeping beauty after the kiss. I imagine what it's like to wake up after 100 years of sleep. In the Ralph Manheim translation of the Grimm's story, "Brier Rose," the princess goes to sleep along with the entire kingdom:

 The moment she felt the prick she fell down on the bed that was in the room and a deep sleep came over her. And her sleep spread to the entire palace. The king and the queen had just come home, and when they entered the great hall they fell asleep and the whole court with them. The horses fell asleep in the stables, the dogs in the courtyard, the pigeons on the roof, and flies on the walls. Even the fire on the hearth stopped flaming and fell asleep, and the roast stopped crackling, and the cook, who was about to pull the kitchen boy's hair because he had done something wrong, let go and fell asleep. And the wind died down, and not a leaf stirred on the trees outside the castle. All around the castle a brier hedge began to grow. Each year it grew higher until in the end it surrounded and covered the whole castle and there was no trace of a castle to be seen, not even the flag on the roof.

I imagine the kiss, what it is like to take that first full awake breath after 100 years. And because it's a kiss, the call of Eros means that every cell is waking up; the entire kingdom is coming back to life. The briar hedge is blooming and falling away.

Often when I invoke this image while dancing, sensation, emotions, my partner, our trajectory, the floor, the room, everything comes into a sharper focus. All the parts of the kingdom become available for this dance, right down to the fire in the hearth. There is the celebration of the wedding that brings the entire realm into balance.

Maybe, just maybe, we have been asleep for 100 years. What does it mean to wake up in this moment?

The most evocative image I've danced with arrived in a remarkable way. In Vienna I was teaching my "feather body exercise." One dancer imagines that every body part is a feather and is feather-light. The 'helper' places a finger under any body part and lifts while the dancer keeps that part as light as a feather so it rises effortlessly.

The exercise ends up with the feather body person on top of the helper while still keeping individual limbs ready to be lifted while almost weightless.

During this exercise one woman sat on the side and was drawing in her sketch pad. I walked over and looked at her drawing. It was clear that she had attempted to draw a body where every body part was a feather. However, what came out was a drawing where every body part looked like labia. I pointed this out to her and we had a good laugh.

Over the next few days I could not get that image out of my mind. So, I decided to invoke this image while dancing. The shift in my body was instant: my parts had more autonomy, ability to listen, and fluidity.

I realized that I could not conjure this image with everyone. If I had to dance at all defensively with a person I would not invoke such a compelling image. But if the dance felt like I could enter with some vulnerability to the moment, this image opened my body and the improvisation to previously unexplored pathways and dynamics.

Over several years the image compounded in my imagination as it went from labia to vulva: each body part is a place of conception, of dryness and wetness, of pleasure, possible violation, the sloughing of the lining, and tumescence. My dancing changed.

D ancing with images, especially over many years, has been one of my greatest teachers. And employing imagery has supported my teaching. In part two of this book in an essay titled, "To the Heart of Feedback," I speak in depth about how teachers can use images to give personal feedback to draw out new worlds of movement in their students.

6

THROWING SALT (WITH GRETCHEN SPIRO)

DANCE AND EMOTION

Gretchen Spiro and Martin Keogh
A post-midnight dance
at the Northern California Contact Jam,
Harbin Hot Springs

Martin:
The evening begins with a new year's ritual
reviewing the months of the year one at a time
My mother's dying and death filled this year
By April I'm cracked open and the tears stream
right through December

Everyone is asked to close their eyes and lay down
"Let me invite you on a trance journey,
to go inside and experience pure energy."
Suddenly language like cotton candy: large and pink,
but after biting into it, there's nothing but air
my teeth begin to hurt
I grow agitated, angry, walk around the room loudly,
finally leave the building

Outside two people are screaming at the moon in
frustration at the hostage situation indoors
The "trance journey" to the "great mother" is followed
by a tedious filling and lighting of ghee lamps,
a ritual that in itself might have been memorable
I feel insulted
I hail the ritual caucus leaders, and open the doors
to my furnace and blast them
I never have opened those portals in public before

Gretchen:
"What led up to this dance? What was your experience?" - you asked
for me to send you something.
i consider making a sculpture of mashed potatoes, coffee grounds
and swizzle sticks.
i write:
The goddamn dawning of the New Year after a year that was
more painful than i ever imagined i could bear. Loving.
Hesitancy. Ceaseless self-interrogation. Challenging the
foundations of my spirit; wondering why i feel so homesick all
the time. My heart cast open. My body quivering in the fear of
change and a terror of leaving. Pain on the underside of my
sternum so great i was questioning whether i should see a doctor.
An attempt to be composed, to Witness the tides of emotions, to
learn compassion and patience. Breathing. Doing my practice.
Doing "the work" with my husband. With myself. Considering
that i might just expect too much. Remembering the vividness of
life and enthusiasm in my veins - and realizing how long it had
been since i felt that regular coursing. "Why am i so merciless
with my pain"

The dance begins

↓ ...Gretchen

Martin... ↓

Several hours into the new year
I come face to face with Gretchen
For a short time, or a long time,
we stand with a few inches between us
A man with a brilliant crimson shawl keeps swooping around us
draping the shawl and pulling it over our shoulders and heads

i see you dancing.
Peter Gabriel sings *The Blood of Eden*
- something about the man, and the woman
i walk up to you,
stand in front of you, and let the person swinging the red scarf
between
us
keep swinging it

I place my palm on the side of Gretchen's head
to say, "This is our dance, Go Away"
she seizes my hand and plunges my fingers into her braids
I clasp my hand and begin to pull
Gretchen looks defiant and inviting
I pull harder and she jumps in the direction I'm pulling
she flies horizontal past my chest
when I no longer can stay ahead of her
I sharply draw my hand down and back
Her body folds in the air like a ribbon,
until she flies in the reverse direction

Throwing Salt (with Gretchen Spiro)

"caught in this curling energy..."
My hair in your fist,
i shatter into my pain.
It hurts, yet nothing hurts like my heart.
i fling myself at you, over and over.
Defiant. Tenacious. Angry.
You lift me by my braids.
"OW!" i cry. But not from this pain.
"More." Dancing takes me.

She slams into the floor
my weight kneeling on her chest and belly
She rolls me off
putting her weight into her hands she kicks her feet
into my chest knocking me backwards
She's standing now, one foot on my chest
the other on my thigh

i have proven my love
held onto it, stretched into the dark recesses
- been working so hard to see into
the dark intricacies
of my nature.
"i am enough" "i am not enough"
i know i could be happier.
i face my grief -
ready to fight, to go to the shadow of sensation.
You are a surrogate for the year's process.
i have surrendered so often, attempted to acquiesce, to witness.
And now i have mercury in my veins.
Poison.
Onto your chest i cast my fear like dice.
Snake eyes.
"Roll again.. ."

Her face is hardened,
she's not joking, and in that
an invitation to discard levity, to dance a brutal frenzy
I toss my torso, throw her off balance
as she descends I roll up to standing
catching her across my thighs
She repeatedly rolls up my torso
I push her down
grab her by the throat

Your eyes are full of madness.
i recognize them, meet them
go out the back door of myself
slamming the door shut, banging the hinges,
cracking the glass.
"See the WITCH of me, - MOTHERFUCKER."
i am not afraid of your hands, your teeth.
Or your ragefearangersadnesspain.

Somewhere deeper than consciousness
our contact sensibilities are intact
I initiate the motion,
into the floor, into the air, across my body,
with my hand and fingers wrapped around her delicate throat

She breaks away
repeatedly hurls her body at me
I can't handle her accelerated weight
Each time I fall under her, or spin her off like a top

No skin, my organs slash open
i dare you to throw the salt. You do.
This body impermanent. Not precious.

We lock arms and press muscle against muscle
until one of us has the leverage and throws the other off
balance to the floor

red red red
Umbilical cord. Hanging rope. Flame.
Blood.
We swim in it, drunken.
Paint scarlet streaks in orange air.
arcs and tones and the space opening
like a great canyon and you fall backwards on the spires.
Crimson rock, layers upon layers.
Dry barren places. Wet stones slippery with dark moss.
There was some odd trust, something that said
"go, go now..." Or never.
Territory where there are no warning signs; danger is implied,
necessary.
We went. Slashing limbs and torso - intertwining, mixing.
A reek of alchemical honesty.
We dangled our secrets over the flames
watched emotions suspend and peel away -
ashes scattering into our eyes,
our sad eyes.

She hurls herself at my outstretched arm
wraps around my hand
I drop with her,
rolling over myself and back to standing
only to find her airborne
and again wrapped around my hand
My arm swings down
swaddled with her body
and swings up until she's perched on my opposite shoulder
briefly

I fall to the floor
She rides the crests of my surfaces all the way down
Fiercely I roll on top of her, and we each try to be
the oil to each other's water,
competing constantly to see who can float roll up to the surface

The open plain. Scorched wheat.
The air hot, inert.
i felt eyes looking at us; i couldn't reassure them, calm them.

The hands don't become fists, nor do they strike as open palms
but every cell in the body is enraged,
wants to bruise the other
We hurl ourselves through space
meeting at first chest to chest
but then fiercely climbing in mid-air
attempting to be the one on top
when we strike the floor

she flings me to the ground, throwing her full weight after me
I fight off the throw when I can, roll with it when I can't

We don't break from the rage that fuels our sinews
Not once do we hit another dancer
We return to locked arms, pushing
bones against bones slowly forcing each other down to our knees
The arms loosen and we fall,
in slow motion into one another and into the floor

i fumble breathless into the crevasse,
Folding into the weeping.
Stillness. A stone at the bottom of the avalanche.
Close my eyes. Seek the mirror. A broken mirror.

"who ARE you who ARE you WHO..."
She flares as a deity in my face.
i have loved her, courted her. Known that
I am her.

stillness now we don't look
My body begins to shudder
with Gretchen's
Our heads fold under a secret tent made from torsos and limbs
We weep, I cry against the depth of violence in myself,
and for Gretchen's trust

                                   there forever, in the no time

Our bodies separate, rise up and each of us sits
we breathe near each other
Is this quiet, or disquiet?

                                   A hand on my forehead
                                   knocks me backwards
                                   back into my too-tight skin

The hands of two invisible people appear
on our foreheads push us apart backwards to the floor
The spell broken
we briefly catch each other's eyes
Is this terror or awe? No words
Gretchen rises swiftly and leaves the room

I try to dance with another
and can't
after this intimacy, it's shameful

I move my body alone

slowly, on the edges of the room
til dawn

After the dance i stand in the shower. i throw low tones and
anguished garble into the water as it fills my mouth. i try to move
forward, to press through time. Unfamiliar songs open the
moments one by one, breath by breath and after a time i turn off
the hot water and don't wince as the cold splashes across my face,
my breasts. i find my towel. Dry my 10 toes. My 2 legs. My crotch.
My back. My chest. My arms. My face. My hair. The outside is
intact. The inside echoes, hollow and alluring.
i make a 4am call to my friend: *"i just needed to talk...wish it wasn't
the damn answering machine...i just had an intense dance...i'm kind of
scared...don't worry, though, i'm ok...i just can't remember who i
am. Bye."*

7

DANCING UNDER DIFFERENT CONSTELLATIONS

TEACHING IN MONTEVIDEO, URUGUAY

(Originally written for the Fulbright Senior Specialist website)

The people of Uruguay have named the different winds that buffet the capital city, Montevideo. The *pampero* brings storms and the *sudestada* brings breezes. *El viento norte,* the hot wind from the north, is also called, *el viento de los locos,* or the crazy-making wind. When the winds switch quickly, they call it *la virazón.* The city sits along the Plate River, and the people here know these winds intimately.

I'm sitting in a courtyard cafe watching flitting goldfish and one lumbering bottom feeder in the center fountain. Looking up, I see layers of clouds conveyed in various directions. I'm about to walk next door to lead a class for the dancers at the National School of Fine Arts at the *Universidad de la Republica*. As I teach we will dance and improvise with the imagery of the winds of this riverside city.

This is my first trip as a Fulbright Senior Specialist. The Fulbright commission has recognized Contact Improvisation in the field of "American Studies." They make available specialists for universities around the world that want to deepen their understanding of American culture and history.

Here, so many miles below the equator, I'm teaching this dance form based on the spontaneous interaction between two people playing with the physical forces that govern their movement. Sometimes it's slow and meditative, and other times it's athletic and acrobatic – the physics are the same wherever I teach, but the metaphors used to convey this form adapt to the local culture and environment.

Warming up in the top floor-dance studio I hear musicians practicing opera, tango, and the sporadic flurry of Beethoven. Occasionally the fragrance of oil paints wafts up from the art classes below. I'm teaching in Spanish here. My voice is lower and not so recognizable to myself. By teaching in another language my material comes out in ways that often surprises me. English is more a language of verbs and Spanish is more imagistic. Where I use the word "core" in English, I use *"medula"* in Spanish. The literal translation of *medula* is "marrow." Asking my students to invoke the image of marrow generates a visceral response – the image leads them to quickly gain access to the strength and mobility found in the body's core.

After class my hosts, Carolina Besuievsky and Florencia Martinelli, take me for a walk along *La Rambla*. This riverside stretch of beaches, walkways and outcroppings runs the length of Montevideo. Teenagers, families, couples, all kinds of people are here – some in bathing suits and some in business suits. Almost every group has a thermos and small gourd called a *mate* from which they drink *yerba mate*, the mildly stimulating tea popular in South America.

I look towards the city and the architectural picture is potluck. Buildings are constructed of brick, stone, concrete, and wood. The roofs are tile, cement and thatched. While this country has just over three million people, the infant mortality rate is lowest, and life expectancy and literacy rates are the highest in South America. Everyone kisses each other's cheeks when they meet.

I am struck by the amount of live music in this culture. I often see people carrying instruments and frequently hear live music in restaurants. On weekends, neighborhoods are filled with the pulsation of drums in preparation for carnival – the evolving tradition passed down by African slaves who were brought here centuries ago.

Most cars are small – I've only seen two SUVs, and pedestrians do *not* have the right of way – today I was grateful for my dancer's reflexes when I leapt out of the way of a turning bus. There is no such thing as lanes – cars weave between each other and I've often disembarked from a taxi with my knuckles blanched white from gripping the seat in front of me. There are horse-drawn carts driven by people who are *humilde* – indigent. They go through the city's garbage and collect the recyclables for their livelihood. Some of the horses are adorned with an elegant or oddball bonnet or fedora.

People here, true to their reputation, have been magnanimous. Patricia Vargas, the Fulbright Program Officer, took me to lunch in the pedestrian mall in the old city. We could hear a familiar sound of Montevideo – doors and windows slamming in the wind. After our table umbrella blew down the street, we settled into the calm of the restaurant's interior. We talked about culture, politics, history, and about our children -- she has a two-year-old and a ten-month-old waiting for her at home.

The meals have been remarkable, particularly the dinners in people's homes where I felt I was immersed in the culture and not skating over it like a tourist. We never ate before 10pm, with 11 being more usual, and once we did not sit down to eat till one in the morning. I'm partial to this lifestyle where the food you prepare you purchase that day from the produce stand, baker, and butcher – all found within a block.

One night we had cheese soufflé at 11:30. The *sudestada* breeze was passing through the dining room. Over dinner, Florencia began to tell me of the days when she was a girl living under the military dictatorship in the 1980's.

I had not realized that Uruguay has its history of incarcerations and disappearances. She spoke quietly about how every citizen was classified as "A", "B", or "C". The "A's" were not seen as a threat and could go about their business as usual. The "B's" were watched and many lost their jobs. People classified as "C" were jailed or disappeared. Florencia's parents were classified as "B". Both were attorneys and her father represented the people who were jailed for their political beliefs. Because the families of the political prisoners often had no money, they would sometimes give Florencia's parents gifts of hand-woven ponchos or other crafts.

I arrived in Uruguay four days after the election of president Taboré Vasquez. This is the country's first-ever socialist government. As of this writing there are left leaning administrations in Uruguay, Argentina, Bolivia, Chile, Venezuela and Brazil. People here are keenly watching Chile because their military has just apologized for the atrocities of the 1980's and a pension has been granted to the survivors.

After our first full week of dancing together, my hosts took me to the countryside near Punto del Este. Uruguayans have a remarkable talent for hanging out. On both days we chatted, ate quail eggs like popcorn, and finally, around 3 pm, someone would ask, "anybody want to go and do something?"

We went to the beach and later toured town. It's a good thing we did not go to the seaside earlier – though Uruguay is one of the

least industrialized nations, it sits squarely under the ozone hole and the sun is brutal. We slathered on 60SPF sunscreen despite being on the beach so late in the day.

Following our weekend respite, I was dropped off in the countryside to catch the bus back to Montevideo. After a long wait I learned the bus had broken down and it was not clear when the next one would arrive.

Sitting by the side of the road, in this country far from home, in this state of not knowing, I found myself gazing at the stars. On this windless night, the Milky Way was so bright it cast a shadow. It had been years since I witnessed a night sky this brilliant. Even the constellations are different in this hemisphere. I reflected on how this dance form has invited me into new cultures and environments. As my senses have been stimulated in new ways, at times I find new doorways opening in my perception, my teaching, and in how I relate to people. I'm extremely grateful that my "work" allows for these experiences.

The bus arrived just before midnight.

During this final week of classes we have investigated the dancing we can do while in the act of falling. There have been shouts of excitement, fear, and glee, as we've worked in the adrenalized moments just before the resolution of a fall. On the last day of working together I could see that each dancer had a newfound trust and connection to themselves and to their partners.

At the end of class a group of students came up to me, and one, in near perfect English, thanked me for my work. She said, "We have been talking, and agree that while we have teachers come here who teach many styles, what makes you different is that you make us feel so good about ourselves." That was the kindest acknowledgment they could have given me.

8

TAKING A STAND (WITH KEITH HENNESSY)

DANCING IN TIMES OF WAR

A conversation
at the Seattle Festival of
Alternative Dance and
Improvisation (SFADI),
Keith Hennessy & Martin Keogh
August 2003

The Activist Urge

Martin: My work as a dancer no longer satisfies my growing need for political action – for being more proactive to make the world a better place. Now that I have a son and three stepsons I feel it's all the more important to do something.

For years I've wanted to be more politically active and haven't found my doorway into that.

Keith: I recognize how the activist urge has more focus and gravity when you have a direct relationship with children and the next generation. Each generation and community get the struggles of their times. So far no one has declared Contact Improvisers to be the new demons, and they are not hanging us in the public square. Historically, people have lived with that kind of conflict.

Martin: I was at a residential Contact jam at Earthdance in Massachusetts with 80 people in 2002. I set up a structured conversation on "the pride and shame of being an American post-9/11." Several folks thanked me for organizing this event, but only a few people showed up. Two of the people who did come gave a harangue about why the U.S. is such a terrible place – and then they left. They didn't want to enter into a conversation.

I was more interested in embracing the paradox: the challenge of balancing our love for our country with our shame for what our country does in the world. It was discouraging that there wasn't more interest. It confirmed a lingering feeling about the Contact community, with its base in individuality and pleasure-seeking, that we are acutely apolitical and apathetic. There are pockets, and you are in one, that are more politically active, but in general, when I travel the country and the world to teach, the individuals in the Contact community are not politically aware or active. I feel this is one of the dark shadows of the Contact dance form.

At ECITE (European Contact Improvisation Teacher's Exchange) in Scotland, there were 80 Contact teachers from 22 countries. We did a score investigating national identity and culture. For the first time in the 19 years of ECITE we took a look at these issues. It turned out that many participants, earlier in their lives, had used their art for political expression, and several had been arrested in political actions. Yet most felt that they are not doing enough now. What I heard many people saying was, "I don't know what to do, I don't know how to take a stand."

Keith: I also feel unsettled within both the improvisational dance world and the circus world with how many people want to do their art and make it a refuge from the chaos of the rest of the world.

Living in the Refuge

Martin: There is something valuable and replenishing about having a refuge. But I think many of us are attempting to live in the refuge, and we are leaving a lot of work that needs to happen undone.

Keith: There are people who are doing meditation and awareness classes in prisons, and the prisoners are feeling like they are experiencing freedom for the first time even though their daily body movements are legislated by timed beepers and guards. They find freedom through some sense of learning to be present. I think this is one of the key things we teach and try to experience in improvisational dance. It has value in that we can take refuge in the moment.

Martin: This idea about refuge keeps knocking around in my head. In Argentina, which already had the biggest Contact community in the world, there are ten jams each week in Buenos Aires, a couple of which are attended by over a hundred people. When the economic and political collapse happened, the Contact community increased dramatically.

I hear from my friends in Argentina that the crisis has made Contact bigger because it is a refuge. There was little money, there was little work, and many of their bank accounts were still frozen. Amidst this, Contact is where people congregate, it is their community. In Israel, it is similar. After the intifada and crackdown started, Contact blossomed and the disparate groups of

Contacters that have existed for many years now dance and organize events together.

Keith: I think that Contact as a refuge in response to political turmoil has two aspects. One is the aspect of escape. But more important is the laboratory aspect, in which Contact - as a life/art dance form - offers tools for releasing the grip of living in fear and tyranny.

During the late '70s and early '80s when 30,000 citizens in Argentina–including activists, artists, teachers, union organizers, and cultural visionaries–were disappeared, there was an attempt to destroy civil society, democracy, and experimentation, even memory. Possibly the huge allure of C.I. in Argentina was, and is, to fill an enormous desire to renew and rediscover touch, contact, collaboration, partnership, sensitivity, and awareness.

Protesting the War

Martin: When it became clear that our country was going to go to war in Iraq against the public opinion of most of the world, something in me woke up and realized that I can't just live in the refuge. I have to DO something. I began to receive hundreds of email petitions and articles – it was overwhelming. The yelling and sloganeering at the marches didn't feel right to me. I felt helpless because I wanted to do something to state my opposition to the war, but didn't know how I could express that. Of course, I would have liked to use my art somehow in that expression. How did you find a way to participate?

Keith: A lot of what we were noticing was that people wanted to go but that they didn't want to go anonymously. So, we went in groups.

On several occasions, someone would put out a call and a lot of people we know, mostly artists, dancers, and a few musicians, would show up wearing white and usually hang back and skip the rally part. When we had enough people, and when the march set out, we would in a sense be our own march within the larger mass of people. We brought our flavor of trying to take peace to heart and not be out there as yet another army.

I remember one occasion when people stated that they wanted to show up and express their grief and rage–we were upset at what was happening. Norman Rutherford and a few other people got these loud reed horns from North Africa and they led the group. There was this loud horn sound and then all kinds of dance activity–mostly flocking scores–happening behind it. We were 40 or 50 people, dancing, singing, and marching together.

Sri Louise, who is also a dancer, has a whole yoga crew–The Underground Yoga Parlor for Self-Realization and Social Justice. They had been going to actions, ignoring the "us vs. Them" politics and putting their sticky mats down in the street and doing a peaceful yoga practice. Beautiful! A couple of times it was known that they would be arrested, and one time when the police came, they were in some posture and they just brought their hands behind their backs with zero resistance. As if to say, "We know what we're doing, we're just going to keep doing yoga, you're not even going to have to ask us to put our hands behind our backs, we'll do it for you." Then Sri got shot with a rubber bullet, and a lot of people said we need to go to the next action wearing helmets to protect ourselves, and I said, "No, we need to go naked."

The next action was way up in San Ramon, and naked wasn't what we ended up doing. We went wearing simple black dresses and we painted our arms from elbow to hand and the lower half of our legs red and we did the whole action barefoot. It was cold and uncomfortable. We had small signs, hanging from a string around our necks, that had a red background with a single emotion painted on each sign–Grief, Rage, Shame, etc. We did a slow "following" score.

There were counter-protesters in SUVs with American flags blaring music and yelling and insulting people. We were silently moving in and out of the spaces between the protesters and counter-protesters. You could feel the protestors calming down around us.

At the big San Francisco protests, the police would handcuff a group of demonstrators and cordon them off to arrest them. There would be a tense energy in the space between the police and the handcuffed group. We would go into that space, where the police would normally not let anyone go, with slow arm movements and mudra-like hand gestures. Yet we had set up this energy where we were moving slowly and singing and decreasing the tension, and found we could move right through. You could feel that we were applying dance skills regarding energy, performance, responding to other's energy, and we were being useful in the situation.

When we went as groups this way, we felt good about participating. Then, when some of us would go to an action alone, we'd immediately drop back into feeling alienated and ineffectual. Part of the alienation was feeling that the people with the microphones seem to know what they're doing, and everyone else is sort of following them around and then feeling non-productive. We might as well go creatively into the street rather than not go at all.

Martin: And what about the folks in your community that didn't want to attend marches?

Keith: Several times we held salons to get people to talk. I held one at the gay/lesbian center. With four days' notice, over 60 people showed up. We put out a call in the email to bring in people who wanted a place to express their feelings about the war. It was beautiful to spend an evening brainstorming about the things that we can do, and what we can do together.

Martin: Did you come up with alternative activities?

Keith: There were people who felt like they were in solidarity with the demonstrators in the streets, yet didn't attend because it was too violent. They were interested in bringing together body-workers and healers to give sessions to people who attended the demonstrations, so they set up spaces for protesters who had been hurt or traumatized.

There were several salons about how to talk to the people in your life who maybe don't have all the information that we have - how to help them get that information, understand it, and believe it. For instance, that the government lied about the weapons of mass destruction. The idea of reaching out one on one, articulating our ideas amongst family and friends and making an effort to discuss the issues together.

There were people who wanted to speak up using ritual and prayer, and one group organized simultaneous "yoga for peace" classes all over the Bay Area. There were about 30 different studios happening on a Sunday two or three weeks after the war started. More mainstream people do yoga, and they see themselves as cultivating some inner peace. These classes were a way to reach this group.

When the war first broke out, a group of us decided to magnify an image that dancer/juggler Frank Olivier had created at an earlier demo, Wearing suits, with real-looking blood dripping down our faces, we went to one of the huge marches and as it came our way, we walked against the flow. We kept saying, "Everything is fine, go home, there is nothing wrong." We did it for two and a half hours.

Martin: And people were just passing by you?

Keith: Yes, and I'm talking about more than 100,000 people that went past us. And a number of times our presence stopped people. We would link hands, and say, "Everything is fine, go home," and people would stop for a while. Then I would say, "Five white guys in suits can stop this many people!" and then people would sort of wake up and join in the theater of it and break us up.

Paradoxical Motivations

Martin: What I'm getting from you is this word "community." Taking a stand in a community is more effective - and less prone to feelings of isolation - than when you try to act alone. And since our's is a dance community, the dance naturally becomes a part of the "stand" we take.

In 1976, I was a student at Stanford University, and my politics were much more important than my studies. I lived in Columbae, a house with the theme of social change through non-violent action. We were re-politicizing the campus, which had not seen protests in several years.

We were the first universitfiy in the country to protest the school's investments in South Africa. We were demanding that the school divest from companies that did business there. During the culminating event of the year, at which point I did political theater in the cafeterias, in the "quad," and at the protests, over three hundred people were in the process of being arrested. I was there with a megaphone getting the protesters to cheer those who were being arrested as they were led away or carried away handcuffed from the occupied administration building to the police vans.

I was suddenly aware of the roles we were all playing in this engagement. To bring attention to that, and hoping the police would treat us more humanely, I said to the crowd: "Let's give a cheer for the police for their role in this human drama." People responded with a huge "Boooooooo!" In that situation, people could not relate to the police as people.

A few days later, I left Stanford in the middle of the third quarter and went on a long, reflective hitchhiking trip across the country. I left because I was disillusioned. I realized how much I loved holding that megaphone, and getting people to lean to the left and lean to the right. Yet I didn't really know all that much about people in South Africa. I had been caught up in my own desire for power. I was disillusioned with the movement, with politics, and with myself.

Yet a few years later, universities across the country were divesting from companies that did business with South Africa, and then Congress voted to follow suit. Then apartheid fell and Nelson Mandela was released and became president. Now I look back and feel like I had a small cell of influence on that, and that I had made a bit of a difference, even if at the time I couldn't see it.

Our motivations can be paradoxical. If there is a way that we could accept paradox, we could involve more people

Keith: I've been thinking a lot about paradox being one of the signs of maturity. Recognition of paradox is a diminishment of innocence. You're both proud and ashamed of being American. You can recognize your privileges as well as your oppressions as an American. Paradoxical ideas are almost never spoken of at demonstrations. If we don't find ways to speak to these paradoxes, there will be fewer people wanting to participate in a full, creative way.

Activism in our Dancing

Keith: When I teach my week-long performance improvisation workshops, I've been trying to have one day focused on political issues. It is slightly awkward to get going, as most people want to be working abstractly and from internal sensations.

I've been setting up an exercise about opposites. You're in physical dialogue with someone else, such that when they go high, you go low; they go horizontal, you keep vertical; they go slow, you go fast; building up a vocabulary about the many ways you can oppose each other.

And then I have people do it alone, as if the dialogue is within them. Without a lot of explanation, people do an embodiment of contradiction, paradox, polarity.

Then, later in the week, I introduce the idea that almost everyone in the room wishes they were more political, but don't know how to go about it. I suggest that if they were aware that they could do it in their art, they would be more likely to engage with political activism. I try to introduce the possibility that they could still have integrity with their aesthetics while using art to explore and address a political situation.

There are a lot of people wondering how to do that, and their first impulse is towards political propaganda, which can be boring or alienating... even offensive or insulting.

One thing I do is sit in a circle with students and we talk about the different wars in the world. We invoke as many places as possible where people are struggling. It creates this big vortex of how bad it is.

Martin: "Wartex."

Keith: Right, a big "wartex." Then I have people start improvising. Many report a feeling of numbness or shutdown. "How can I get present to that and perform it or improvise with it?" I encourage people to bring their own personal feelings and ideas into the room - into their gestures and actions. James Hillman speaks of "entertaining an idea" and I invite folks to do just that - to not try to solve a problem or even to know what they're trying to say. Dance, especially improvised movement and performance, is useful for researching and expressing complex interactions of thought and feeling. I prefer performance that is simultaneously sad and angry, awkward and graceful, confident and reflective.

I've also been talking to people about the sense of relationship between the art we make and the ancestors.

Martin: Our ancestors?

Keith: Let me say "our" or "the" ancestors. In theater, we often think of the audience as the fourth wall. Michael Meade has been challenging me to re-think this - to imagine the audience as a semi-circle and that the ancestors complete the circle, with the performer in the middle. The idea is that when you step on stage to perform, you are standing between the two worlds of the living and the dead - being an oracle between these two worlds.

I'm trying to build a communal and larger spiritual context for what we do, so that people will stop being so individual and understand that the performance is not just about them and their intuition and presence. This focus on the individual leads to alienation rather than solidarity, community, and caring about others. This becomes a long-term project around building community and relationships to the future.

Martin: I like that phrase "building a relationship to the future." This allows our political and performance work to not be about instant gratification.

Keith: Yes, and we are not in that long-term project if we are seeking refuge all the time. I feel like saying "Come on, people!" It is another thing I do in my work; I try to increase people's tolerance for pain.

Martin: I guess "tolerance for sensation" is how I would phrase it.

Keith: No, I want them to tolerate pain. I want them to sit in it when something hurts and have the realization that it isn't the end of the world.

It's one of the things I work on continuously in my teaching, to encourage people not to give up so easily and not to sit out. The idea that as soon as something hurts at all, it's abusive.

I believe that if you want to feel connected to the people of the world, then find something you care enough about and work hard at it. Working hard and dedicating yourself is your ticket to breaking the cycle of alienation; not by withdrawing from work or challenges that are difficult.

Standing Up

Martin: If we take a stand, we are attempting to lean on the culture so that the culture will move to a different set of beliefs. Keith, you have chosen a lifestyle that is substantially outside the mainstream. Don't you worry that by being on the outside, you don't have an effect on the people in the middle?

Keith: I don't necessarily think my stance is about trying to get everyone to join me. I want more people to express their opinions and to participate in a radically democratic project called human cooperation and life.

I see it as having a position, and the culture comes to you. It's like creating a gravity. Because of what you're doing and the way you're doing it, you pull the people to you or attract them to your idea. You can affect the conversation, even if you're in the minority.

Martin: So you're taking a stand, not to lean against, but to attract or pull towards your world of thinking. But by taking a stand far on the fringe, you attract fewer people.

Keith: I work on the idea that what we need is more people working on the edge rather than the center. That by stretching the edges of the culture, you give more room to everybody. Even if you say my strategy is about creating gravity, I'm not trying to get people to necessarily join my circle, but at the point that they turn away from the TV, they'll find something on the way between that and me that will suit them better.

I'm working with a "multiple-front" political theory, that if all these people are doing something around the edges, then there are plenty of places for people to go in different directions. We don't need more centers; we need more edges.

Martin: I like the kinesthetic sense of what you're saying; if you take a stand on the edge and a few people move toward you, then there is more room in the center.

And if you take a stand right where you are now, you don't have to make big changes in your life to take that stand. I feel this is essential to bring more dancers into the political arena. To let them know they don't have to make a huge step from where they are right now to be active. They simply need to stand up.

———

To contact Keith Hennessy: jkeithhennessy@gmail.com / Keith's website: http://circozero.org

Thanks to Jill Cooper for transcribing the tapes of this conversation and for doing the final edit

This conversation with Keith was, in part, what led me to create the book: *Hope Beneath Our Feet: Restoring Our Place in the Natural World*. You can get information about all my books at martinkeogh.com/books

9

THE 38 GIFTS OF CONTACT IMPROVISATION

A LOVE LETTER

D ear C.I.,

Thank you for:

- a network of companions and collaborators all over the world
- for resisting definition, codification and doctrine
- for not making us dress up
- for the practitioners who bring the discipline of language to their research
- for not being trendy
- for a strong and supple body
- for some fine performances, and a few really bad ones
- for the adrenelinnnnnnnnne

Thank you for:

- the generosity of the people who teach this form
- for the challenge of dancing with people of all different abilities

- for not having to learn steps
- for being fertile ground for metaphor
- tor being a dance that welcomes regional, temporal and personal variations
- for the friends, colleagues and lovers
- for not being dependent on charismatic leaders
- for always being an incomplete form–so people get to complete it with themselves

Thank you for:

- the ability to intimately connect with people who do not speak my language
- for being a compassionate mirror of who I am in all my relationships
- for the range of touching and being touched
- for deepening our capacity for pleasure
- for teaching us to allow one moment to be the seed of the next moment
- for helping us become permeable to life
- for the absence of maps
- for the time we get to inhabit our reptilian brains

Thank you for:

- the reverence dancing with men and the rapture dancing with women
- for being my living, my support, my lively-hood
- for not having certifications, belts, diplomas, ranks, and hazing initiations
- for the laughter
- for getting to be around (and around) such wonderful bodies
- for bringing us closer to the corporeal pulse of heart,

intestines, and lymph
- for the increasing awareness of the physical forces that govern our movement and lives
- for such pleasantly earned rest and sleep

Thank you for:

- inspiring humility in me by how inclusive and magnanimous you are
- for the moments (I love these moments) when curiosity spills over into fascination
- for being so accessible but also for not being simple
- for being such a spontaneous yet consistent partner
- for being so magnanimous with our aging bodies
- for keeping us so close to the worlds of paradox and mystery

**Contact Improvisation,
we go back 38 years,
and I love you. Martin**

10

CAT'S PAUSE AND BARE FEAT

IS CONTACT IMPROVISATION PERFORMABLE?

"A craftsman always knows the result of his labor, while the artist never does."

— *W. H. Auden*

The Zoo

I was a consultant to Eszter Gál who single-handedly organized the 14th annual ECITE (European Contact Improvisation Teacher's Exchange) in Budapest, Hungary, in 2000. She took many of my suggestions, but there was one piece of advice I'm glad she rejected.

She told me that for the performance evening she planned a four-hour marathon. Since we had over 120 Contact Improvisation teachers together, she wanted to give everyone a chance to perform—some more than once.

I was aghast.

I told her that people don't have the capacity to take in more than an hour of Contact Improvisation. I pleaded with her to make it shorter and allow everyone to leave hungry for more. She looked at me kindly, thanked me, and said that in this case, she was going to do it her way.

Eszter rented the Artus/Fono Budai Music house, a factory converted into a cultural center. She turned every nook and cranny of the various buildings and outdoor walkways and plazas into performance spaces. People migrated from area to area like treasure hunters discovering what was around the next corner. There was an outdoor stage and two indoor stages. People danced in trees and suspended from fences. People performed between the tables in the café. Duets were happening on the sink tops in the public bathrooms. In the gallery that held an exhibition of remarkable dance photos by Thomas Häntzschel, there was an ongoing round-robin. On a descending outdoor walkway between the indoor and outdoor theaters, lit only by the full moon, a dozen nude bodies were curled up like boulders strewn down the path, peeking out from the surrounding foliage. One meandered through this landscape of glistening, moonlit forms.

On the outdoor stage, something might start at any time, a planned meeting or a spontaneous "pickup company." At one indoor stage with full stage lighting, there were three rounds of one-hour performances with various dance artists each hour.

The evening served to skew people's perception of performance and life. If people are dancing on fences and in trees, what does that mean about how I move through my day? If people are performing while we sit drinking tea discussing Hungary's history with Romania, how does that influence our conversation? If at any time I can move to another performance, another perspective, or begin to perform myself, what does that do to my role as spectator?

Eszter was courageous in her vision and her trust in the performers to understand the potential of the various spaces.

The last performance on one of the indoor stages was a contact duet that continues to reverberate in me years later. Rick Nodine from the U.S.A. and Jovair Longo from Brazil were the finale of the evening. The stage was back-lit as they ran in together. Their silhouettes ran fast from one corner of the stage to another. Without a pause, they would turn at a corner and keep running in step and close by one another. The sound of their feet falling in sync made a compelling rhythm. Suddenly Rick fell and Jovair fell over him. Instantly they were back up and running again. Then came repeated tumbles. Sometimes they fell side by side and sometimes one would pitch or vault or plunge over or onto the other and into the floor. They continued until they were visibly tired and their hard breathing joined the sound of their footsteps.

Finally, clearly exhausted, they dropped to their backs breathing hard. As their breath settled, the two back-lit bodies began to breathe in sync with each other. We could see the rise and fall of their diaphragms and the sweat gleaming on their faces. There was a sense that as their breath calmed and joined, we too joined them in their breathing. They were in tune with each other and had tuned us to them.

Slowly, almost simultaneously, they began to move. They paced the dance and took us with them—sometimes in a slow lucid rolling of the contact point around their bodies, and sometimes with an effervescent lobbing of each other into the air and to the floor and back up again. As the improvisation built, the stage lights came up to full. Their relationship was filled with curiosity, tenderness, affection, edginess, near confrontations, little and big assists, and a robust physicality that left us tingling and ready for more when they finished.

That sultry evening in Budapest, Rick and Jovair brought us their dance, one you might see them do at a contact jam. With the tuning that came from the running and breathing, they invited the audience's complete involvement as they put their dance on stage.

They were performing Contact Improvisation. Many people question whether C.I. is a performable dance form. When I see duets like this, which live on in my body and imagination for decades, I'm convinced that it is.

It's perplexing that some of the most engaging dancing I see happens at jams rather than in performances. Often the same dancers who have such a solid connection at a jam abandon their Contact faculties when in front of an audience. They seem to forget about something as basic as rolling the contact point. They don't venture off-balance. They leave their skills of discovery in the moment for more controlled movement as they shape and compose the dance. They lose the sensation as they focus on the design.

Rick and Jovair brought to their dance all the sensational aspects of C.I. and let us in on them.

I confess that in the past I've not been a good audience member. My judgmental mind would run rampant. I'd often envy the fact that it was not me on stage. For years I just didn't go to performances. Finally, I developed a score for being an audience member that made it enjoyable for me. I go with a pen and a pad of paper. After a period of time in which I've been absorbed and unselfconscious, I write down what just happened. In this way, I've been able to articulate those elements that pull me into a performance. My aesthetic has become clearer. And at those shows where my attention drifts, I have pen and paper to write down my flights of fancy.

When I first started dancing in 1979, Contact Improvisation was at an apex. I had discovered the vocation of my dream, and I threw myself into it completely. At the time, there were many Contact Improvisation dance companies in the United States and Canada, including ReUnion, Men Working, Catpoto, Mangrove, Free Lance, Contactworks, Freefall, Mirage, and Fulcrum. By 1981, many of these groups had disbanded, and C.I. performances in the San Francisco Bay Area where I lived went fallow for the next few years.

When C.I. began an upswing again in the late eighties (one that continues to this day), the form had changed. Many dancers were answering the question "Is C.I. a performance form or just a participatory dance?" by bringing more of a compositional awareness to their performances. Rather than allowing the physical forces to guide the improvisation, people seemed more interested in how the improvisation guided the physical forces. I miss the former aesthetic.

Ann Cooper Albright, who teaches C.I. at Oberlin College, once told me that she feels that ballet and modern dance go outward and penetrate and colonize space, while in C.I., it's the other way around—space colonizes and penetrates the dancers. C.I. is introverted, and it's difficult to communicate to an audience the internal landscape of sensation and responsiveness of the performers. This is one of the greatest challenges of putting C.I. on stage: How do we communicate the rich tapestry of sensation, of choices and discoveries being made, when most of these are internal experiences?

Over the years, I've come to believe that two elements are crucial here. One is the environment—the context you invite the audience into—and the other is the tuning—how you tune the audience into your world.

When people come into a theater with a proscenium stage, there is an immediate expectation and desire to be entertained, to be dominated by the experience. For Contact Improvisation, the performers need to give the audience the tools to shift to another perspective from which to experience the performance. Doing a lecture-demonstration or seating people right on the stage are ways of changing this expectation. Brenton Cheng, a dancer in San Francisco, looks for ways to tune the audience into the mindset that they would take to the zoo. You don't expect the animals to perform for you, you simply observe them as they go about their business, following their own rules, being who they are. This zoo environment was created in the ECITE performances in Budapest.

There are myriad ways of tuning an audience. I've seen many performers start with a slow arriving into their own sensations and movements as a way to tune themselves and the audience.

Rick and Jovair tuned their audience by running in step and inviting us to breathe with them. By beginning with high energy, they created an anticipation that we would see more high-energy athletic dancing later, and they fulfilled their promise several times over.

I've seen performers create a lot of chaos with many bodies in erratic motion and then clear out to reveal a single duet in the space. Out of the chaos came something crystalline, and our curiosity was awakened to how the duet would continue to reveal this order.

Once, in a performance workshop, two dancers entered and faced each other with just a few inches separating their bodies. They looked into each other's eyes with this condensed space between them. With their feet planted, they let the tops of their bodies spiral back and forth around each other like two snakes. The eye contact and the closeness of their lips made this a charged beginning, filled with erotic possibilities. Their improvisation grew from there and took me with them in the suspense that comes with the presence of Eros. As audience members, we created narratives of the making or breaking of relationships, seductions, falling-outs, and reconciliations.

What comes out of these beginnings is a tuning of my perspective and expectation. Suddenly I am brought into the process of discovery, into the dance, into the sensation; feeling the choices being made. A conduit opens into the inner landscape of the dancers and I readily go with them into the unfolding of the improvisation.

A t the zoo, we are fascinated by the unselfconscious interaction between the animals. Is this fascination a hint to what works well in a Contact performance? At the zoo, what do most people want to see? I've watched large groups of spectators stand engrossed as two rams repeatedly backed up and then hurtled themselves at each other with their horns colliding like thunder. I've heard people cheer two horses on as they nip and sniff each other in their pre-copulation dance. It's no wonder that when two dancers exude sexual chemistry or the potential for violence, it gets our attention.

Jess Curtis and Stephanie Maher began a piece by standing in front of each other using these phrases: "Hit me"; "I don't want to hit you"; "I want you to hit me"; "Make me hit you." Then one slaps the other's face. Then the other slaps back. This goes back and forth until a contact dance grows out of it. The audience became viscerally alert, wanting to see where this improvisation goes next.

When I watch Ray Chung and Chris Aiken perform together, I feel like I'm at the performance zoo. When they dance, they are performing as themselves rather than putting on personas. They are willing to make eye contact with each other and the audience, sometimes with some acknowledgment, like a smile, that helps put me on their side. I'm often delighted by how clearly they enjoy themselves.

I like to see their handsome bodies in motion, these skillful movers in control and out of control. It's exhilarating to see the moments when their restrained physicality bursts into vigorous movement. And I'm engaged in the moments when their extreme physicality makes me imagine the danger that exists, that one or the other might get hurt. And I'm calmed and relieved when they take an earned stillness that comes after a lot of activity. Both Ray and Chris have mastered the skills of contact, and when they are in performance, they use these skills generously.

The Feast

The dance that excites me the most is based primarily in the basic skills of Contact Improvisation, in the body's response to the physical forces—gravity, inertia, centrifugal force, etc. This is the meat and potatoes of Contact Improvisation.

To cleave to these skills, Ray Chung and I often use a performance score that we call Dance On/Dance Off. We develop our contact duet offstage and then enter the stage dancing in contact. We end by exiting the stage dancing together. This keeps us connected to the form, and it gives the audience the image that they are seeing a slice of our dance, a dance that has been going on—and will continue—for a long time.

What can be added to the meat of Contact Improvisation are the spices that our animal natures evoke when we come into relationship with one another. Adding a dash of spice can be just the right thing to make the play of the physical forces come alive for an audience.

There are many spices, but for the sake of this essay I want to differentiate three of them: space/time (salt), narrative (garlic), and emotion (chili pepper).

When I'm in the audience and I'm given a bowl of spice without the meat and potatoes—when it shows too much narrative or contrived emotional expression or arbitrary composing of the space and the timing—it makes me grimace. But a pinch here and a smidgen there can make the performance tasty.

The salt of improvisation—the awareness of space/time—is by far the most in danger of overuse in contact. By becoming overly aware of how the dancers are relating to the space around them or to rhythmical qualities, Contacters often lose their inner body focus and can lose track of their partner.

But a dish without salt can taste flat. Eszter Gál is one example of bringing the right dash of salt to her Contact Improvising. When she dances, the physical forces are at work and our attention is drawn to her body. We can also see her relationship to the edges of the stage, to the negative space between her and her partner, and to us. While connected to the dance she's having with her partner, Eszter lightly salts the relationship with phrasing, contrasting stillness with motion and playing with tempo and repetition. And her use of space/time awareness often leads to dances that end dynamically with the dancers, the space, and the audience all connected.

Movement that has strong intention and specificity is the clove of *garlic* that creates imagery and narrative in the mind's eye of the audience.

Cinzia Gloekler is a dancer skilled at bringing narrative into her improvisation. Though not literal, each motion seems pregnant with meaning. When Cinzia looks into space, whether it's the space between her and her partner or out past the horizon, the space comes alive because she appears to be seeing something. Stories are created by the relationship of her hands, which way she faces, her limbs that sometimes seem to have lives of their own, her sudden changes of velocity. I've seen her create an instant narrative by simply walking in step with someone, then falling behind, breaking away, or speeding up.

When we are on stage, there are many relationships going on— our relationship to our dance partner, to the audience, to what we are doing, to performing itself. We have feelings about these things. A person who can spice with emotion, or what I call chili pepper, knows how to let their feelings be seen. By revealing what's going on inside, the power of weather systems moves through the performers and the theater.

Sabine Fabie and Gretchen Spiro are dancers who include their emotional bodies in their dancing. Their enjoyment of dancing shines on their faces and in their playfulness, and their pleasure is contagious. As their emotions change, the dynamics change— from tender to aggressive, clingy, ecstatic, afraid; the list could go on and on. Their emotions bring power to their dancing.

Including the emotional palette in the dance adds tangible dynamics to the quality of contact. When I'm angry, my hand lands on my partner's shoulder differently than when I'm feeling bored or playful or fearful. The right amount of chili pepper can make moments more charged and engaging because the audience can feel their own emotional bodies through the dance.

I saw a trio that had a wonderful balance of the physical skills of contact and spices at CI25, the twenty-fifth anniversary celebration of Contact Improvisation at Oberlin College in 1997.

This Contact event, with almost 240 Contacters from 19 countries, had a particular but not unusual irony. In the two nights of performances, there were only two pieces that I would call Contact Improvisation. One was Ray's and my performance of the Dance On/Dance Off score. The other was a trio with Nancy Stark Smith, Karen Nelson, and Andrew Harwood.

The three entered the stage together and each began to slowly, gently try to be in between the other two. This physical act immediately created a narrative because they each had the same goal, yet it was not possible for them all to succeed at once. Starting with this clear simple task immediately tuned the audience in to their experience and sense of discovery.

They tried sliding in, going in underneath, becoming the trickster by suddenly changing directions to go around and sneak in the other way. And then they began to move away and to jump into the center. Out of this came sudden perches, slides, and carries. Gasps came from the audience as the dancer's bodies seemed to suspend in the air for longer than was physically possible. There were the unexpected surprises of all three jumping at each other at once, or one being knocked over by the other two. The bodies would keep falling out and the energy would constantly be recycled back into the center. It was like one of them was fuel, one was oxygen, and one was heat; they each kept igniting the others to a hotter flame. The dance built into a fast, risky, airborne, quick fall–quick rise crescendo. And then it ended near its peak.

Their task created two narratives: one filled with humor that made us laugh out loud, the other filled with potential danger that kept us on the edge of our seats. In their lightly spiced, physical Contact Improvisation, there was a searing beauty that lives in me to this day, as only Contact Improvisation can.

This piece reinforced for me that spices don't work on their own. One generally does not sit down to eat salt or garlic or chili peppers. But subtly added to the core body state and the pure engagement of Contact Improvisation, the performance can become a feast of the senses and imagination.

It's a challenge to trust the basic principles of Contact Improvisation when in front of an audience. But dancing in a suitable environment and tuning the dancers with the audience can allow us to do the dance our bodies know. Adding the spice of relationship can bring the dance up to the level of art.

———————

Endnote: "Cat's Pause and Bare Feat" was the title of an evening of Contact Improvisation that Riccardo Morrison and I presented in 1981.

11

SKILLS OF 'LABBING'

Contact Improvisation is researched through jams, workshops, festivals, and preparing for performance. Because this is a research-based dance form, one valuable format is the "lab." Dancers gather in open or invitational groups and enter their inquiry through dancing, talk and reflection.

In my first year dancing I studied with 19 different teachers. In my second year I kept taking some classes but spent about ten hours a week in the studio labbing with different individuals. We would dance and then work with our curiosities that arose. This was a natural next step in my maturation as a dancer and teacher. Labbing has continued as a practice through the decades.

I enjoy the challenge of being invited into a studio with a teacher who says, 'I want to teach X, and I don't know how to do it.' Leigh Hollowgrass was preparing her class for the West Coast Contact Festival and invited me to join her to lab her class material. She wondered if it was possible to fly downwards onto someone. If a person was dancing with someone who has gone to the floor from their wheelchair, or anyone in a low post, how can the able-bodied dancer still get time airborne?

We worked on this and found that one could leave the floor and fly down to someone who is on all fours if they arrived spinning so the weight went into the centrifugal force rather than into the post. We worked backwards from this discovery to create small steps to arrive at the outcome. Leigh taught a skillful class where almost everyone was able to get an experience of this.

For years as I danced, I wondered how to invite/encourage people through my dancing to trust entering their backspace with me. I tried many techniques: tapping them with my head, pushing with my upper back and then releasing, touching the top of their head; nothing seemed to consistently work. I brought this question to a lab group and someone said, "Have you tried putting a hand on their hip bone." Standing back to back I tried putting a hand on my partner's hip. The person immediately relaxed back into the support. This lab question, which I had struggled with on my own for years, was figured out in two minutes and we moved on to another question.

At the first Contact festival in Buenos Aires we did a fishbowl teacher's lab where participants proposed questions and then witnessed the teachers in the act of labbing those questions. We labbed several skills by request. Then we labbed a few of the teacher's questions including one of my own: Can a person fly onto someone who is already over the edge of their balance and falling to the floor?

Slowly teachers peeled off until it was just Daniela Schwartz and myself grappling with this question. We progressed to the point where Dani was curving her body with tone and doing a banana fall to the floor from standing. I joined her with my hands. Then I joined with more of my body. And eventually, I flew into her as she did her long-edged fall with me glued to her in the descent. It was as if one body was banana falling and receiving the floor's support. While this opportunity does not show up often in the dance, my body now has an increased confidence to engage with people who are off balance.

In San Miguel de Allende I convened a labbing group that met five days a week for over three years. The core group included Leilani Weis, Daniela Schwartz, Viet Fuentes, Paula Zacharias, and Nancy Franco. Because of the constancy and extended time-frame we deepened our physical and emotional trust with one another which allowed us to engage in more complex and edgy inquiries.

We worked with sloughing, where we would pick someone up belly to chest so they would completely relax in our arms. We would then release them suddenly so they would stay relaxed and free fall to the floor with minimal engagement. Over the years we tried this from a bench, from a table, and then from two tables stacked on each other to see how a person could stay relaxed in a fall even from dizzying heights. We got to the point where we could hold the person upside down with their head touching the floor and they could free fall slough from an inverted position. (Do NOT try this at home!)

We spent a year investigating "rides on the fly." We wanted to move past those lifts where you wink at your partner and then fly a rehearsed pathway up to their shoulder or hip. We investigated a state of availability that allowed rides to appear out of the moment by following curvatures, rising momentum, entering the under-arcs, and falling over fulcrums into the rides. While we were in this investigation our jams were filled with the exhilarating, spontaneous acrobatics that can arise during my favorite dances in Contact Improvisation.

We worked physical questions and emotional questions. We worked clothed and nude. And we asked questions about witnessing the form that led us to performing every few weeks.

Proposals could be half baked, and things did not need to work in the end. We had permission to try wild ideas. Our ideas were free to metamorphose into something altogether different than the initial impulse. We got to find our edges and move from there. The chemistry of this lab group invited a range and depth of investigation that informs us two decades later.

One time we went too far.

I came in with a burning question. I noticed that when I danced and saw a person flying towards me, I had an emotional upwelling. When I saw someone launch in my direction this surge of emotion would give me the capability to deal with their weight when it arrived. I identified the emotion as anger and I wondered if this would be useful for smaller people to manage the weight of bigger bodies.

I had us think of situations that made us angry and then we flew into each other. I brought in sticks and had us break them and then fly into each other. We tried pushing our partner and then flying into them but none of these created the desired effect.

I don't remember who had the next idea. We stood in front of our partner, and with permission, we slapped our collaborator in the face and then launched our body in their direction. The result was extraordinary. The smallest people in the room were heli-coptering the largest people around their shoulders. Being hit in the face created such a torrent of sheer sinewy strength that for a moment we almost had superhuman powers.

While this was illuminating and informational our group was an emotional mess for a week. We had to do a lot of slow confidence building to get back to some sense of balance and harmony and trust. While it was startling to us as a group, I don't regret going over that line. It demonstrated that there was a limit within which we knew we could safely investigate.

I 'm fascinated by the set of skills that grease the wheels of a successful lab. In my longer workshops, I teach these labbing skills. This started because I kept hearing of injuries in labs as a result of people addressing questions for which they were not adequately warmed up.

When we do labs in the context of a workshop I make sure people are warmed up for any eventuality. This includes activities that allow us to:

- read the nuance of sensation
- get the core muscles fired up
- dance at a heightened heart rate

Once these three areas are covered we are ready to enter the unknown.

For the first round of labs I give the topic. Often we begin with an "alternative pathways" lab where people identify their patterned pathways and then find alternatives. We normally work in groups of three or four.

The next round of labs each person brings their personal question they are grappling with. The group gives time and focus to the question of each member.

The next round, and most challenging lab, is for the group to together come up with a question they all want to tackle. I enjoy the moment when I see the light bulb ignite over everyone in a group because a single idea has them all excited to engage.

I give this lab guidance before we break into groups:

- The key to a good lab is generosity. Generosity with listening, with your knowledge, with your presence.
- Everyone's desires are important: it's up to the talkative people to make sure the quiet ones get to bring out their contribution.
- Empty the cup: there might be someone who knows something about the question already. Let them empty the cup by telling or showing the group their knowledge. Then move on from there.
- Notice lab envy. Notice your envy of other labs in the room.
- Give your lab a title: When you can agree on a title you have a focus: "Invitations that bring greater sensitivity." "The mechanics of little lifts." "Allowing instability to invite the unexpected."
- Balance talking, movement research and dancing.
- If you are looking for your lab question, or if you have a lab question but need more information: start with dancing.
- In labs we don't necessarily find the "answer" but hopefully get a deeper understanding of the question.
- In the labs where each person brings their personal question, it can call for some humility. We are venturing into an area where we feel unfinished. The group can acknowledge the courage of this action.
- We sometimes jump at the simple answer to release tension. Welcome the discomfort and stay longer in the unresolved. This allows for more surprising discoveries to arise.

I normally give one hour for people to work together (a little longer for the personal lab questions). The lab groups then bring their findings to the entire class. Some offer a report on what they found, or better still, give a demonstration or a demonstration with a report. This might be of one discovery or they can show a medley of discoveries. Another option is they can lead the group in a simple exercise to demonstrate one of their findings.

L abbing is an invaluable way to deepen our investigation of the dance. The format of labbing works especially well in communities that don't have the critical mass for a weekly jam. It only takes two people to have a lab.

At the end of my workshops I often give homework. Sometimes this includes: finding a partner or small group and lab weekly for six months to a year.

12

DANCING DEEPER STILL

QUALITIES OF A SEASONED CONTACT IMPROVISATION
DANCER

I reached a period of boredom with my habitual movement patterns after one year of dancing – it seemed that most moves, most choices, I had reworked hundreds of times. During a month-long intensive with the Mangrove C.I. dance company, I was sitting with three of the teachers and lamenting how bored I was with the repetition within my dance.

"This is a good development," John Lefan said, almost beaming. Freddie Long said, "Boredom is a sign you have awareness of your patterns and this is the first step in moving past them to something new." And I remember Byron Brown adding, "one definition of an advanced Contact dancer is someone who has numerous cycles of boredom under their belt."

I'm fascinated by the qualities that seasoned Contact dancers bring to the form. And I'm beguiled by the challenge of articulating those qualities.

A t the ImPulsTanz Festival in Vienna, perhaps the largest and most prestigious dance festival in the world, I'm regularly perplexed by how many dancers join "advanced" Contact Improvisation workshops who have not taken even a single class in the form. For the most part, these are exceptionally well-trained contemporary dancers and human specimens. I'm doubtful they would sign up for an advanced ballet or kathak class with no previous experience. Yet with the organic quality of movement in C.I. they presume they already have the needed skills.

While the students come in ready to 'partner', the excess tone in their bodies make it challenging to listen to and converse with another body. They find skillful well-trodden pathways in and out of the floor, but are ill equipped to fall freely without hurting themselves or their partner. It is often challenging for them to let go of composing a dance and instead allow it to be discovered.

I've discussed this with several C.I. teachers who have passed through ImPulsTanz. Most of us end up teaching Contact fundamentals regardless of the posted level of the workshop.

P erhaps identifying the necessary fundamentals for an unimpeded inquiry is more important than identifying the qualities of an advanced dancer. What constitutes the foundational propositions and skills of the form – those elements we need in place before we can venture further?

Here is the language that Chris Aiken and Angie Hauser use to help people self-select into their advanced workshops:

 Experience level of participants:

We are accepting applications from advanced level C.I. dancers. We appreciate the challenge inherent in this kind of self-assessment, and offer the following criteria, to help clarify. As an advanced C.I. dancer, you should be able to:

- Take weight
- Fall safely from different levels
- Follow the point of contact
- Move upside down, be comfortable with disorientation
- Be able to modulate the physical tone of your body in relation to your partner and the demands of the dancing
- Be committed to being emotionally clear and present while dancing
- Accept responsibility for your own safety

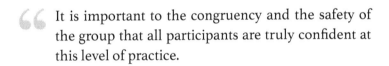 It is important to the congruency and the safety of the group that all participants are truly confident at this level of practice.

And here is language Nancy Stark Smith uses for her January month-long training for returning students:

Although levels in C.I. are difficult to assess, your C.I. practice should comfortably include: fluency with falling safely from any level, rolling, weight taking and giving, being upside down, dancing with disorientation, following a point of physical contact, working with subtlety (and exertion), and improvising in physical contact.

Both these descriptions are precise listings of refine-able fundamental skills and capacities. Once learned, they allow us to move together safely in a dynamic physical conversation. From here our research can get increasingly wild and refined

I t remains a perennial issue how we as practitioners and teachers create a criterion for advanced work. Most people agree there is no single scale upon which we can rank dancers who research Contact Improvisation. There are many, if not innumerable benchmarks upon which to measure ability. Once we have the fundamentals of what it takes to move together in close proximity without a guiding plan, the continuing investigation seems to come down to personal inclination.

Steve Paxton said that "survivability" was a major criterion for who he invited to participate in the first group to explore his ideas that became Contact Improvisation. He wanted folks with the resilience and ability to survive what he was going to throw at them. Daniel Lepkoff, a teacher and a member of that original group says (from CQ, May 2008: Contact Improvisation: A Question?):

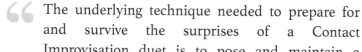 The underlying technique needed to prepare for and survive the surprises of a Contact Improvisation duet is to pose and maintain a question:

- What is going on when I move?
- Where is my center?
- Where is down?
- What surfaces of my skin are being touched or touching?
- Which of these surfaces offers support?
- Where do I think I am going?
- Where am I able to go?

- What am I not aware of? ... and so on

While the first group to dance C.I. were invited because they were athletes and dancers considered able to 'survive it'; we now teach the skills of survivability. This has opened the form to be inclusive of an extensive range of participants. The form is, by nature, magnanimous.

However, in all its magnanimity, I've come to feel it is crucial to have forums where we investigate beyond the fundamentals. By dancing at the edges of what we already know, then the dance evolves and flourishes, both personally and collectively.

It is here where the dance gets interesting.

H ere is one way I differentiate newcomers from seasoned dancers. When a person begins Contact Improvisation it's similar to a city installing its first subway lines, with only a few stops along the route. People reach the terminus station and then need to turn back.

It's the same with dancing. As a beginner continues to dance, they build more stations before they need to turn back. Then they develop new lines and transfer stations.

What I've noticed with seasoned C.I. dancers is that they have practically no terminus stations. They may choose to turn back at any time but they don't have to. It's a choice – a choice most often exercised when faced with a wall or another duet in the way. The seasoned dancer has enough cycles of boredom, and moving beyond their patterns, that they develop a near infinite metro (or U-Bahn, or Tube, or Underground, depending on the city and country). The follow-through can be near boundless, and by cleaving to continuity the seasoned dancer can progressively ride themselves into newfound pathways,

The fundamentals allow us to dance safely in physical conversation together. Then what each of us decides to research and identify as "advanced" is a reflection of our personal proclivities. For myself, I'm fond of asking **IF/THEN** questions: **IF** this foundation is available, **THEN** what can we do?

- **IF** we know we can pass weight through our body to the floor, **THEN** we know we can surf other bodies along the floor
- **IF** we can pass the weight of our partner through the structure of our bones, **THEN** we can carry people bigger than ourselves
- **IF** we can fall from greater and greater heights, **THEN** we can develop the skills of flight
- **IF** we can enter a spiral **THEN** we can offer many relatable places in our body for our partner to respond to
- **IF** we have no terminus stations, what **THEN**?

Below are some abilities and skills organized according to my proclivities. If people have elements in the first list, they can then play with qualities in the second. If fluent in the second list, they then have the foundation to research the qualities in the third list.

Savvy in the fundamentals, an "advanced beginner" has:

- skills of body perception/ trust in their proprioception / awareness of where they are in space
- ability to modulate tone. Moves expansively, colorfully, but with a feeling of little mass, like cotton candy

- ease with pathways to/from the floor, alone and together
- ability to pass weight through their tissue and bones to the floor without the need to 'muscle' it
- the facility to listen through touch and the ability to follow a point of contact
- equal comfort in choosing to introduce the front side of the body as the backside into contact
- precision with weight, on and through the body of the partner
- comfort using the hands as landing gear
- ease refusing weight, a lift, or touch. Can slough off, get out of the way, or discard what is unwelcome
- an increasing capacity for the unresolved and the awkward
- an ability to continue in the physical conversation during moments of disorientation

An "intermediate" dancer with fluency in these abilities has:

- a body that is organized and released, has a pliant strength, is supple and resilient
- limbs and head that move autonomously from one another
- legs that are free and can empty and hips that can disengage when the person leaves the ground
- comfort accepting invitations in the dance by almost instantly unweighting a point of support. This includes, while on the floor, unweighting the core by delegating weight out to the limbs
- the freedom to not automatically ground through their feet as the dance is free to move through the room
- a head that easily leaves a vertical orientation to the room— entering spherical dancing
- a new ability; the invitations that used to be delivered by

the hands can now be given from anywhere on the body
(the ribs become fingers!) The dance goes from being
manipulative to being more consensual

- the capacity to read the space and the floor through their
  partner's body even when not in physical contact
- a use of mirrors to get spatial information rather than to
  see how the dancer looks
- the skill to find recuperation inside exertion
- an ability to save themselves when falling from height
- the ability to see and move into the backspace
- a sense of sourcing the improvisation from follow
  through rather than frequently introducing new ideas
- a comfort giving up custody of their center to a mutual
  center. A capacity to give up one's ideas of the current
  trajectory

**A "seasoned" dancer, beginning to investigate at these
edges, has:**

- begun to allow any point of the body to be ready, at any
  moment, to initiate in any direction, at any velocity
- an expanded ability to send invitations that used to be
  given through touch but now can be broadcast and
  received through the space between bodies
- many relatable places in their own body offering
  multiple points of engagement: I call this poly-centric
  dancing
- the capacity to dance with a lucid touch. Their partner
  can feel not only the touch, but also feel the partner
  feeling the touch
- a visceral understanding of the spiral; falling AND
  spiraling into the backspace
- the ability to make the space around themselves

tangible. To not rely solely on their partner, they project past themselves to get support from space itself

- an understanding of how to fall into the spontaneous acrobatics of the form (rather than the "wink, wink, I'm about to fly into your shoulder" lift)
- a virtuosity born of entering dynamic movement without knowing how it will resolve itself
- a presence that dilates time by leaving something behind (often by spiraling) so that newfound impulses can be sourced from the past, the present or somewhere ahead along the present trajectory
- the awareness of not dancing their skills so much as dancing with their partner: this is why they have the ability to dance with people of all levels of experience

The original group to investigate Contact Improvisation practiced three skills that became the original frame within which to meet to dance. They worked with Aikido rolls, the 'small dance' of meditating on the act of standing, and the exercise of leaping through space at one another.

Over the nearly five decades since that original group met, a myriad of skills has been developed and added to the frame. To name a few that were not in the original investigation that we now take for granted: pouring weight; work on low and high posts; pathways into the ground and into the air; and the basic skill of surfing. These and an abundance of other skills have been developed since the beginning days.

After so many skills have been amassed, the question becomes how do we not fatten the frame so we are dancing skills superimposed on skills? As we advance our research, how do we remember the original proposition of the form, and allow the enlarging frame of skills and abilities to give us a more abundant territory within which to meet a partner in a state of curiosity?

Nearly a half century after its birth, Contact Improvisation continues to evolve, spread, and influence other movement forms. It is important for the development of Contact Improvisation to research with seasoned practitioners who are actively investigating at the edges. When seasoned dancers work within a group where we don't have to be concerned with self-preservation, where we don't need to dance defensively, where we don't hold back, then we may be moving at the edges of the form itself.

Here are a few venues where seasoned dancers research together:

- European Contact Improvisation Teacher's Exchange (ECITE, in a different country each year)
- C.I. Ground Research (at Earthdance)
- The teacher meetings that lead up to Contact festivals
- Advanced level workshops
- And one of my favorites: regular invitational or open labs

This essay evolved out of the thoughtful, probing, and sometimes furious responses I received to a blog post I posted at martinkeogh.com

You can join the conversation at:
martinkeogh.com/what-are-the-qualities-of-an-advanced-contact-improvisation-dancer-part-one/

Puedes unirte a la conversación en Español en:
http://martinkeogh.com/spanish-version-cuales-son-las-cualidades-de-un-bailarin-avanzado-de-contact-improvisacion/

13

MOMENTS OF RAPTURE
DANCING CONTACT IMPROVISATION

The Instruments

Who is the luckiest in this whole orchestra?
The reed.
Its mouth touches your lips to learn music.

All reeds, sugarcane especially, think only
of this chance. They sway in the canebrakes,
free in the many ways they dance.

Without you the instruments would die.
One sits close beside you. Another takes a long kiss.
The tambourine begs, touch my skin so I may be
*   myself.*

Let me feel you enter each limb, bone by bone,
so that which died last night can be whole today.

Why live some soberer way, and feel you ebbing out?
I won't do it.

Either give me enough wine or leave me alone,
now that I know how it is
to be with you in a constant conversation.

— Rumi (translated by Coleman Barks)

We pitch out through the tops of our heads, leaving our feet behind, we fall together, both rolling into each other's bodies as we descend, not foreseeing who will be on top when we reach the floor.

I dance with the image that I am a river and you are the banks of my river. I don't know what's downstream. I let that come. If the shores get narrower I move faster, if the banks get wider I flow slowly into the tributary. If I encounter a boulder I can flow around it or go under it and pick it up, or go over it and get lifted. I'm constantly being drawn. At the same time I know I am also the shores to your river and you, too, don't know what is around the next bend.

The backs of our hands meet. We follow their nomadic pathway between us and through the room.

You are a stranger at the jam. I will never learn your name. Our authentic, spontaneous contact entails surrendering our needs to gain or profit from this interaction. We relinquish a desired result or outcome. Contact is the crossroads where we meet, where information and goods are exchanged. Contact is the market-place, the watering hole, it is where we allow ourselves to be affected and where our strengths and limitations are challenged, encouraged, and tested. Authentic, spontaneous contact is about entering the exchange and flow, willing to bargain our perceptions and actions without fear of loss or promise of resolution.

I'm on all fours. You are standing next to me and using my back like a trampoline to fall into me and be bounced back up to standing, only to fall into me again.

Old friend, I remember the pathways even after all these years. It's familiar, I know this dance because we have had decades of traversing together. We've indelibly imbedded who we are into each other's cells and synapses–what we like, where our inviolable edges are. And here we are years later dancing in the thin air of central Mexico, finding ourselves airborne and flying and bellowing with our remembered delight.

Dancing with you is like dancing with myself. You're big. I roll up your standing back to your shoulders and I keep rolling towards your head and circle from shoulder to shoulder like a helicopter blade twirling.

With you I like to sweat and feel my lungs at their full capacity. And be pushed and push back. And whoop. I feel my skin blossom with the contact of your skin into beauty. And when I dance I do feel beautiful – strong, resilient, creative, courageous, sensitive, human. Our dance makes me feel I'm reaching something whole.

We run through the room, and with one hand on each other's shoulder you are airborne for every five steps I take. And when you come down, I find myself leaning through my arm on your shoulder, spinning feet out perpendicular to you, flying around in circles.

You are tiny standing next to me, yet when you dance you become large, so substantial.

I dance Contact with you because I love the thrill. Falling off center and knowing that I have to have the abilities to save myself when I need to. Living and playing with the physical forces as we two individuals negotiate our time together. The thrill of living in the instability of human interaction.

I *jump through space flying horizontally to alight on your chest. Rather than stand there and catch me, you jump to join me, pivoting my flying body in the air and we turn inside out as we fall soundlessly to the ever-waiting ground.*

I dance Contact with you to feel like an animal, to lose all thought, to stop plotting the future. To live in what this moment brings, to be in the hunt, the adrenals at full throttle here in the Savannah, the lion having just come into view.

W*e are standing head to head feeling the slow sway up through our bodies from our soles.*

I live with this ideal–like a poet who wants to write with the profusion and profundity of Shakespeare–I dance with the ideal of occupying the same space as you. Not only sharing the same time, but to be where your body is in this moment. How do I do this? Do I push my way in? Do I become porous and blend with your cells? Do I find the smallest portal possible and pour my fluid self through that opening?

I don't know yet, but I keep looking year after year, decade after decade for that consummation in the dance. Sometimes it feels sexual. More often it feels sacred, like an ultimate merging and dissolution into the immeasurable.

I'm standing knees bent. *You are arched back, your shoulder at my hip. I realize that if I jump from here I will take you up with me and you will be standing with me on your shoulder. I know your ability to take care of yourself anywhere, anytime. I leap. To our mutual surprise you are running through the room with me on top, the wind in my face.*

Our dance becomes the speculum through which life is experienced viscerally, beyond thoughts of empire building, closer to the corporeal pulse of heart and intestines and lymph and our blood ties to the seasons and tides.

A*s we run through the room together, we take turns flying into the under-arc up to each other's hips.*

We depart from the archetypal, from living by ideals, and being champions of virtue; it's no longer the battles between the gods. For all that, as in the mythological worlds, our dance is generous. We are awarded an abundance of images, encounters and sensational touch.

W*e are repeatedly falling into each other, surprising ourselves each time with where we end up. Sometimes swooning into rolling, sometimes falling up into hugging the narrowest cliff edge of support for a ride that extends into the next fall.*

I dance Contact for the sheer fluid pleasure of moving with other bodies, feeling their spirit as they pour their weight into mine, as I pour myself into them. The scent of my dance partners, seeing their eyes as we acknowledge the humanity of the other; the feeling that this is not just some avocation, some social dance, but a form of re-wiring, of finding ourselves with a mature capacity for ongoing joy.

Y*ou stand almost a head taller than me. I feel safe taking off airborne in your direction, not knowing what will come of it.*

I dance Contact with you so I can feel what it's like to soar like a hawk, dive as an otter, tussle with lion cubs, slime like a slug, hover like a humming bird, be pursued like a deer. So I can feel what it's like to bear down on prey, sleep on a rock after shedding my skin, break out of my pupa to dry, and spread my wings for the very first time.

W*e repeatedly bump into each other until we fall down in a laughing heap.*

I dance to know the stories of my partners. What do their tendons tell me, their willingness to support, to trick, to arrive, to contain? And what story are we creating together, now?

W*e are back to back, feeling the support of the other.*

One of the more painful aspects of this form is the constant admission that I don't know–I don't have it all figured out. Sometimes it's boring, I'm not satisfied, I want more, I want less, I feel like I'm not meeting you well, I'd rather be in another dance. You're too sweaty, seem distracted, you're too manipulative.

You are the mirror of my existence; the same unconscious willfulness I bring to the dance I bring to my life. With you, with every partner, I get to see a tangible and sometimes startling reflection of how I live all my relationships.

I get in this rock tumbler with you, knock around with you, so that my sharp edges soften. So the gemstones hidden inside will begin to peak through.

W e are both twirling around our individual centers. Sometimes our butts or hands meet as we come around.

Contact Improvisation is like an artesian well; the water keeps coming once it's found. Some days one has to find the source of the spring again, but once unearthed, it soothes, nourishes, enlightens.

After mirroring our judgements, our desires, our limitations, the dance brings into focus a quiet place. After cajoling, massaging, challenging us to accept who we are as we are, a deeper still rises up. The earth breathing us with no need for will.

There comes a moment of acceptance, of living in the current texture of sensation and interaction and motion, except that we are in the eye of the hurricane, at ease, allowing the rest to swirl.

W e push, grab, tackle each other. We cradle and assist.

I dance Contact because I'm a sexual being. Dancing with men makes me proud to be a man. Feeling the strength of my partners, their sweat as we push up against each other makes me know that I have a place to stand in this world.

And when I dance with women, smell their scents, I get to experience a dance that comes from rapture. I get to feel the cells coming alive, to know that I'm part of the link between generations – that my sexuality is connected to something greater than the personal.

And while I go home to the One woman, when I dance I can feel my attraction to the many.

W*e are surfing each other's bodies across the floor.*
We dance Contact because the form is unfinished. It's not a choreography that we rely on, rather it's a series of principles that needs you and I to perfect it. We are the completion.

W*e move to stillness, bellies down to the floor.*
It's late at night at the jam in Potsdam. We have danced long and hard and we are both on empty.

It's like we've hiked a strenuous day and finally dropped ourselves to the ground. After a while on this mountaintop our eyes focus in the grass near to our faces. We notice the world is moving. Flowers that are smaller than pin heads come into view, and here is an ecosystem of 4, 6, 100-legged creatures going about their day of collecting food, mating, building homes, crawling, burrowing, waiting.

In our dance, when we slow down, become myopic, we discover worlds of aliveness. Moving only a few inches brings in whole new ecosystems to delve into. Feeling the contact point; what is here? Can I slow down enough to feel your breath, your pulse, your story? With these newly disclosed details our dance continues enlivened once again.

W e are rolling the point of contact up the switchbacks of each other's bodies.

I dance with you because I haven't answered the question: Why? Why am I alive? Why are we here, embodied? Why do we have to die?

I dance with you so life's moments become tangible; our tissue merging gives reason, gives sense enough. I might not have the answers, but I palpably dance the questions.

A gain, as we dance, our faces are wet with tears.

When we do Contact what we do is so simple. We meet physically and see where we go. You are a puzzle of movement patterns and possibilities that meets my collection of pathways and desires. Where do we go together? What is our dance this moment of this day?

Yet tucked into that beguiling simplicity are worlds of untamed emotion, raw face-to-face contact, moments of heart-rending tenderness, and the exhilaration of flights between constellations.

When we dance nothing is hidden. There are moments of clear mirrored reflection, sometimes flattering, sometimes startling. For another breath of our short lives we live awake, dancing towards the shimmer when the curtain goes down one last time.

14

OLD GROWTH

AN UNFETTERED MEDITATION ON DANCING WHILE AGING

I used to roar into the dance studio and begin by jumping off the walls – becoming sweaty and energetic and frothy. Then I would slow down and shift into sensation. Now, in my 60's, I slide into the studio and start slow, steeping in the ale and gradually working up to the froth.

The words "young" and "old" have never made sense to me. But I appreciate now the notion of aging, of time passing and changes in the body and outlook. I live with more physical limitations than ten years ago, when I had more than twenty years ago. I used to identify so much with my physical prowess and agility. As those have lessened I've had to adjust how I see myself. And I've had to pull back my desires – I'll probably never do that back handspring again.

The elder dancers whom I respect have each blazed their own way. The image from the tales of King Arthur comes to mind – "Every Knight shall go out and enter the forest where there is no trail." Dancers like Remy Charlip – in his elegance he's brought the designers eye from his costume design into the dance. Anna Halpern has ridden the wave of what's popular, been shame-

lessly a decade ahead of others. Bill T. Jones has brought the raw
edge of human interaction and the emotional body into his
work. Steve Paxton rolled a pebble and then got out of the way
for the avalanche that followed. They've each blazed their
own way.

I met the blazing dancer, Akram Kahn in Vienna after seeing his
one-man show DESH. We talked about aging as dancers. He said
that it used to take him 45 minutes to warm up for the show. Now
it takes a full three hours.

When I look at my wrinkles, the accumulated scars, the skin that
doesn't pop back right away – a reality sinks in. When I started
dancing in my early 20's, I felt immortal, convinced I would never
grow old... or conservative. I hitchhiked 25 thousand miles with
the full knowledge that I would be safe, and I was.

I don't hitchhike cross-country anymore – though I still hitchhike
locally on occasion to put myself back into that sense of time –
standing, not knowing who will stop, or if it will be three minutes
or three hours. I don't sleep on the floor anymore, or futons when
I can help it. I prefer a mattress – a pillow-top mattress. And, oh
god – I'm more conservative. I support a family. I need to care for
myself so that I can care for them. Though politically I'm more
progressive than ever.

The lost resiliency means that now there is no room for error. If I
overdo it I pay for my mistakes over a protracted period of time.
Known pathways are safer even if less interesting. What is most
important is getting myself into a state of flow so I can take risks.
Getting into a flow state is the most important prerequisite to
having fulfilling dances... even if it does take three hours.

As I'm less reckless with my physicality, I have also become less
reckless and more disciplined with my ideas and language. Now
when I teach I rarely toss out ideas just to see the effect they have

on people. I hone more so that what I do convey has the benefit of my experience.

My view of teaching has evolved. I used to believe I needed to be at the center of everything to teach a good class. As my body has changed, I don't demonstrate or partner as much as I used to. "Teaching" is about showing our students the ways we have found – whereas "cultivating" dancers is about helping them blaze their own trails. Now the role of "mentor" is more important. I see myself nurturing future dancers and performers, and cultivating communities of dancers. The paradox is that more I focus on others and entire communities the more recognition I receive.

When the up and coming, the young hotshot dancers, vault and spring through the studio – I sometimes feel a tinge of envy and loss. Mostly, they keep me fit – I'm moved by them to stay in shape and creatively engaged so that I continue to have something to offer – so the treasury continues to overflow. Contact Improvisation is a magnanimous form. It allows people to dance and teach as they age. The form is not about someone's abilities, it's about modeling the inquiry and investigation into what's possible.

When I spend time with people my age I notice the tendency for us to kvetch about our ailments. Incessantly. The limitations and pain of aging are real and talking about them discharges some of the built-up frustration. But talked over to an extreme and the ailments become the person. So, I have a rule: I'll talk about my ailments no more than six minutes in any given day. That honors them and allows me to be more than my collection of limitations. Hopefully much more.

On one hand, I'm romantic about the idea of getting older. Rather than considering myself older, I like to think I have more rings in my tree. And then I say – what kind of bullshit is that? It sucks to get older. The body becomes more limited, organs and muscles fall apart, we see more of the insides of hospitals, we lose energy, courage, our abilities. Aging is about loss.

We know the boat is sinking and it all comes down to the attitude we bring to that descent. Do we go down numb, or screaming, or singing? I miss not worrying about my health, the late nights, the excess. I'm glad I fully lived my youth. What is it that King Arthur's Knights seek anyway? The Holy Grail – the fountain of youth, of everlasting life. Don't most of us, somewhere in ourselves, want that? Isn't that why people head out in the first place to enter the woods where there's no trail? While I feel like I have found my grail through my work, that I've created something that will live past my own life, I want to be young... damn it.

I remember being in my 20's and having a sense of invincibility. I was going to live forever and change the world to boot. I cannot say that now. Talking about aging is humbling – it demands confronting that indelible piece of everyone's life called mortality. I will, sooner or later, die.

I love my life, and love life more each year. I feel mostly good about the choices I've made along the way. I've been passionate, truthful, and I've spent my life being true to my muse rather than popular culture. I don't want life to end – I want to see how history unfolds – that of the world, of my family, and my own.

My body has given me a great life; I don't want it to end in a slow, painful breakdown. "Aging gracefully," is a concept I've heard about. I believe it has something to do with acceptance. And then there's Dylan Thomas in his poem to his father – "Do not go gentle into that good night... Rage, rage against the dying of the light..."

My fear for the earth and humanity grows with each passing year. I look out the window of my study. I see trees. It's a quiet suburban neighborhood, with trails into the forest at the end of the block. We are in walking distance from the center of town. We have two fireplaces and an above-ground pool in a big yard.

We have the American dream. We have our castle and grounds. We live in a safe, wonderful place. But then I travel and read the news and "out there" the world is a frightful place filled with suffering, environmental decline, and injustice. What have I done to change any of this? What am I doing now? If I were to tell the truth right now I would say that as I age I'm most afraid of the world that I'm leaving my children.

When I was a teenager we were told our generation was the one that could make the difference – that it was in our hands. God knows we tried, and the world is still a fucked-up place. I want my children to have the opportunities to live at the edges of their potentials and creativity and not at the edge of their personal and global survival. I feel regret that I haven't done more to make a difference. Then the other voice comes in – this energy I'm putting into regret I could be putting into making a difference right now...

One morning in my 50's I picked up a bag of concrete that had hardened. I did everything right – got low, pulled the bag to my center, lifted from my legs – and still my back went into a spasm that felt like I was being speared for shish kabob.

I immediately laid down on an ice pack with my legs up. The next day I was worse, and the following day worse again. I wept because I couldn't put on my own pants and I didn't want to ask for help. My wife took me to the hospital where I was given anti-inflammatories, anti-spasmodics, painkillers, and an MRI. I was told that I absolutely must not pick up anything, including my toddler or his toys.

There was good news and bad news in the MRI results. I had no blown-out disks – I can keep dancing. But I have degenerative disk disease, or premature "old man's back". The MRI report included lines like: "*There is a congenitally slightly narrow lumbar canal due to congenitally short pedicles.*"

Since my injury I have not been visualizing myself dancing as much – I used to regularly imagine dances which kept my body in a warmed-up state. Now, the thought of dancing can seem far away from the act of dancing.

When I do dance now, each dance feels like I've received an 11th hour reprieve from the governor. I've been saved! It feels so enlivening to dance. With each duet I savor the exhilaration, the personal unfolding, and the joy of relating to other people this way. I've become re-committed to finding new pathways so that I can dance even when the body grows less able. I want to do the work now, to put myself on a trajectory that keeps me dancing, and experiencing the rapture of Contact Improvisation.

But I am afraid – not so much that aging will keep me from dancing – but that I'll lose my livelihood. I'm passionate about teaching people to dance. It allows me to travel and see the world and meet people, and bring gifts to their lives. If I don't teach how will I support my family with even half as much fulfillment and delight? The thought of a 9-5 fills me with terror. That is not what I want to model for our children. I want them to see their father creatively engaged and being rewarded, not for his toil, but for his development and creativity and connection to a community.

I remember a panel of professional dancers talking about money and aging. The subject created a storm of anxiety. One dancer, Keriac said that when she could no longer work, her retirement insurance policy would be to take her own life. This stunned a lot of us. Later, she confessed that while she thought this for years, she could no longer could commit suicide because it would be too wounding for her now-grown daughter. She was in anguish about what to do, as she was closing in on her retirement years.

It saddens me that our culture offers little support for the arts. It makes it such a struggle to go forward and blaze – especially when we have to consider details like healthcare and retirement. But on the other hand, I see in countries, where there is more funding for the arts, a certain dampening of the artistic spirit. When you live in a cycle of getting a grant to live on for half the year, and receiving unemployment the other half, there is a certain indignity that accompanies this lifestyle. And yet, when there is little support for dance and the arts, there is a certain hardening of the spirit just to persevere.

The body has its losses that need to be grieved, but there is another loss that comes from living in a youth focused culture. I know, as a man, I only feel a sliver of this. I've heard from many older women that when a woman loses her looks there is a way in which she is not seen; she's looked over, not consulted. The attention goes to the young. If an older woman dancer is not in her role as "master teacher" she has to work hard to be seen and noticed.

I've made a practice of watching older athletes as they compete. People in their 70's and 80's playing tennis, basketball, volleyball, and other sports. I sit at the edge of the court and watch them with a question – what do I need to do so that I can dance full out when I'm their age? What steps can I take now to be on that trajectory?

I've noticed in older athletes, that their ribcages can freeze up and this limitation leads to less mobility throughout. So part of my training is to have attention on an increasingly released ribcage. I consider this my practice, my "dojo" work.

I'm often struck by the vitality and glow with which these athletes leave the court. I've sat in on numerous conversations where they grumble about their current ailments. This is often accompanied by their gratitude for ibuprofen for sore muscles, and herbal concoctions for aching joints. I listen carefully. My intention is to join this clan.

I still take pleasure in adrenalized dances where I sometimes find myself moving with my head below my pelvis, my feet somewhere up in the air, not quite knowing what will come next. But along with this pleasure I recognize I have less resiliency and less capacity for recklessness. To safely have adrenalized dances I'm finding that I need to dance with less muscling. Being *ready* for this kind of yielding and potentially high-energy dancing means being willing to expend less effort and will.

Rather than use muscle when I'm dancing with someone who brings a lot of vitality to the dance, I'm trying to develop a body that is porous, like a living sponge in the sea. The strong currents move the sponge but can also pass through the permeable interior.

I'm surprised that my investigation so far into long-term dancing has not suggested more control, but a body that is more awake to the possibilities of the effortlessness of abandon.

A s I age, it's easier to be still. My capacity for noticing details and nuance increases. I can sit in nature and be alone for longer periods. I'm less driven to be creative, to entertain, to receive adulation. I can lie down and observe a square foot of forest floor, seeing layers upon layers of life, with less self-consciousness.

I'm less driven by my hormones. While I sometimes miss the energy that the amplified libido brought into my life, I don't feel as compelled by them now. I love my sexuality and I'm glad that I've had a wonderful canvas to express it on. Now, I'm less driven, and the dissolution in lovemaking is more encompassing.

When I'm dancing I bring four decades of body investigation that informs the movement. When I'm in a duet I might not be as recklessly acrobatic, but I can create a sense of listening in my body that is contagious.

I miss the ability to do full splits and fall from great heights. What I don't miss is the self-doubt and chatter that used to rankle me part of the time. I'm not saying that my flexibility is completely gone, and certainly not saying the chatter is all gone, but both have diminished over the years.

I believe that we lose 1% of our physical abilities each year. However, we have the possibility to gain 1% more awareness of nuance each year. The loss is automatic. The gain of nuance needs cultivation. The question becomes do we choose to give the attention needed to have this added superpower?

W hat about legacy? The dance is ephemeral. When a person creates a movie or a piece of art, it goes into the world accompanied with a name in the credits, or painted into the corner of the canvas. Each dance dies as it's born and only sends out a diminishing ripple of what it once was. A dance might change us, and the resonance might live on, but it is not signed. My legacy carries on through my writing, and somewhat through my teaching, but even these are fleeting.

We sometimes hear about the beauties of old age – but I've noticed that the old age that is beautiful, is the one a person has been preparing for by living a beautiful life. Each one of us, whatever our years, is right now preparing for our old age. The beauty and reach of our questions in the end, determines the beauty and reach of our lives.

PART II

TEACHING RESEARCH NOTES

FOUND PEARLS

15

INTRODUCTION

FOUND PEARLS

There are almost as many teaching styles in Contact Improvisation as there are teachers. We have so much to learn from one another.

Eighty-one Contact teachers from twenty countries attended ECITE (European Contact Improvisation Teachers Exchange: 2005) in Viljandi, Estonia. The group was split into smaller co-teaching groups that worked together every morning for the week. My co-teaching group represented eleven nationalities and I was one of only two native English speakers.

Like all yearly ECITE's, this group collectively had decades of diverse teaching experience. During this event, I facilitated a structure called "Sand Grains Into Pearls." Someone asks a question about teaching – some ongoing irritant, a sand grain in their life as a teacher. If someone in the group has knowledge or experience with that issue, a pearl for that sand grain, they speak it or demonstrate it. Often, many pearls are offered.

In this group we had questions like, "How do you teach smaller dancers to lift big dancers?" "What do you do when you have a student who everyone flees from when you say, 'find a partner'?" "When you have a sexually predatory student in your classes, what actions do you take?" "How do you deal with the student who is routinely instructing their partners?"

When teachers gather at exchanges like ECITE, there is an abundance of knowledge and experience, combined with the generosity inherent in our dance.

This section of 'Found Pearls' is not a "how-to guide" for teachers. Rather, here you will find teaching research notes gathered from events like ECITE, from my own teaching, and from late-night phone conversations with teachers around the world.

I hope teachers of the form (and teachers in general) and those who are considering teaching, find a few treasures here that are useful in their exploration of transmitting the principles of Contact Improvisation.

16

WHO CAN TEACH CONTACT IMPROVISATION?

K nowing when you are ready to teach

Who can teach Contact Improvisation? There is no licensing body. No degrees or black belts are handed out. Nobody with a magic wand glorifies us with their blessing.

How do we know when we are ready? Since I see us as teaching and modeling our *inquiry,* rather than a set of techniques, I feel anyone who is in an active and committed investigation into the form can teach.

If somebody knows the alphabet from A to P, they can teach it to P. If they are honest with themselves and their students, and don't try to teach T, U and V, they will teach a safe dance class, especially since the first ten or so letters of the alphabet are about learning to soften and be safe.

It's a matter of each person teaching at their level of investigation. Students learn from the teachers who put themselves in a state of inquiry and then transmit that state.

W ho decides?

The marketplace has a way of deciding who will teach. When a person decides to hang up their shingle and call themselves a teacher, do students show up, and do they return? Do festivals invite them to teach?

M entoring students to be teachers

I'm seeing more teachers actively mentor their students into teaching roles. They invite students to lead warm-ups and assist as assistant teachers. These invitations are creating an informal system of mentoring, where the investigations of both student and teacher get enlivened. The younger, more athletic students who show up alive with passion for the form help to keep their mentors on their physical and creative toes.

I regularly invite particularly engaged students to assist me. During class, I sometimes take my assistant aside and ask, "What would you do next?", "What does this group need?" Their responses often change my trajectory with the group.

Once, I asked my assistant where we should go, and he replied, "Lead us in one of those things that sneak us into dancing without us being aware of it." Another time, my assistant said, "I see all the pelvises apart: We need to get them together." I asked how she would get this to happen. Her response was so applicable I had her teach the next section. This mentoring supports the form.

As a teacher, one objective is for my students to surpass me.

F inding a mentor

Now to be contrary: So, you want someone to mentor you?

There is no easy way to break this news to you – there is *no* mentor. There is only the fantasy of *the* mentor. You will have to become the teacher you desire.

And if you feel you have found a mentor, rather than love the mentor, love what the mentor loves. This will lead to substantially less disappointment when you reach the level where it comes time for them to take the leap off their pedestal.

17

INITIAL CONTACT

G eography of the dance studio
Walking into a new dance studio I see a large space with a wide-open floor. Yet, I know that every space has invisible lines of demarcation that divide the room. These lines will help shepherd the incoming dancers to particular locations.

There are regions where people go to remain hidden, areas where they go to be seen, and places that welcome interaction with others. As I will talk about later, some studios have specific hot spots where injuries are more likely to occur. Dance studios have hidden geographies that affect our work.

If there is a seating area or windows where people can see in, there will likely be a moat right in front where fewer people dance. Next to this is often an area for the more extroverted dancers; farthest away from the viewing area will be places to be less visible and also more intimate.

A dance studio with mirrors will have a similar psychological geography. Teachers of traditional dance forms often place them-selves in front of the mirrors (or the sound system). This becomes the "front" of the room. The skilled students gather next and the back is where you go to not be seen. To upend this layout, I usually begin class by teaching from the side of the room, opposite the "front".

If there are several people watching a class and a moat begins to grow in front of them, I might ask that they space themselves around the room to lessen the feeling of dancing with spectators (unless we are working on performance).

There are locations in a room where emotion can be expressed and held with greater ease and safety. This is often farthest from the moat. I hold my check-in circles here to take advantage of the support that we receive from the room itself.

It is imperative for me to notice those parts of the studio where my eyes or body rarely go. This way, I can be aware of and teach to everyone present.

The geography of the dance studio is like the geography of the body; we have places we won't look to, places to hide, and body parts that like to show off and seek attention. By becoming aware of, and getting into all the parts of the studio, by discovering the room's sphericality, our awareness can open, and the same can occur in the bodies dancing in the room.

C onsciously entering a new sense of time

I used to arrive in the studio before anyone and take down the clock. Taking the clock off the wall allows our time to be more pliable. But then I noticed it was helpful if the students observed the action of reaching up and removing the time piece, as it allows them to recognize that we are entering a suppler sense of time.

Rituals for arriving

Teachers frequently have a ritual to connect with the dance space. This helps prepare the teacher and sanctify the space. They might:

- Sweep the floor
- Air out the room
- Meditate
- Warm up into dancing
- Touch all the walls
- Go over the name list
- Set up flowers or candles or a shrine
- Walk the ambit, the entire circumference of the room

These rituals can be done before students arrive, and some are good to be witnessed by some or all of the students.

Acknowledging the work it takes to get into the room

I learned a lesson from Ann Aronov about how people arrive on the first day. It can take a lot of effort to get through the door, and it often helps to acknowledge that effort in order for the students to fully arrive. At the beginning of a workshop or intensive, she says something like, "You've done the hard work by getting here – you made the decision, carved out the time, paid the money, and got yourself into the room. Now the hard work is done, and the rest is about ease, like riding a bicycle downhill."

I see faces soften, shoulders drop, and hear people's exhalations when their effort has been acknowledged.

The opening circle

To help people get into the room, I often have people say their names, a favorite comfort food, and show one of their sleeping positions. The favorite food awakens the senses and brings awareness to the abdomen. Showing the sleeping position invites the relaxing pre-sleep breath that leads to a sense of ease. The sleeping position is an intimate detail that most people find easy to divulge.

Other possibilities during an opening circle after they say their names:

- If you could be an animal for a day, what animal would it be?
- What piece of clothing, footwear, or jewelry makes you most feel like yourself?
- Show us a part of your body that is drawing your attention today.

This serves several purposes. On the most basic level, it allows us to attach the name to something about the person. This structure allows people to be seen and heard. Some individuals can't partake in any learning until they feel seen by the group. This helps.

As people show their body part, most of the group feels that part in their own body, so the warmup has begun. This also invites people to acknowledge vulnerable places in their body that need extra care and attention as they dance.

It also allows me, as a teacher, to recognize who the kinesthetic learners are and who the visual learners are by what each person does with their eyes and bodies when looking for the body part they will name.

Honoring those that have come before

A major resource is the act of summoning what I've learned from my past teachers and dance partners. Something alchemical appears in the act of invoking and honoring one's elders and sources into the room. When you name your teachers, it creates a lineage. It connects what we are doing today, in this place, to a larger context, to the people researching through time, and in different parts of the world. When you name your teachers, it links your students to the transmission and gives them more responsibility in their investigation. This also models humility and respect.

Invoking mentors also brings them into the room for their support. This allows me to stretch my teaching style. And if we invoke someone who has died, it brings a reminder of our mortality and a poignancy into the room and into the work.

Invoking our mortality can be a reminder to the teacher and the students of many things. One reminder is that life is too short to hold back for fear of looking foolish.

Stories that are too big to hold

Sometimes, we do something in our teaching, and we don't know why. It took years to figure out why sometimes I like to start workshops with stories like this one:

 While living at the Empty Gate Zen Center in Berkeley, I heard two quantum physicists interviewing each other on the radio. They were talking about how much space there is in each atom. It is VAST.

They said, if we removed all the space from each atom in every man, woman, and child on the entire planet, the mass left over would fit inside a single peanut shell. It would be an exceptionally heavy peanut, but we would ALL fit inside ONE shell.

One physicist asked the other, "If we are this spacious in our atoms, how come we can't simply pass through one another?" His colleague said, "If you have a fishing net, no matter how large the holes are between the strings, you can't pass one net through the other without breaking it."

I now realize the efficacy of this image of spacious atoms. Students arrive to a first class filled with varying proportions of expectation, resistance, and desire. This mixture has a daunting potential to hinder the student being present and receptive.

Some teachers welcome people into the room and deal with this blend of anticipation by leading the group to the subtlest details of sensation, so that all else is forgotten. Some teachers use humor, and others get students interacting right away.

Another way to work with this initial class moment is to offer an image too big to hold in one's imagination. My experience is that the anticipation that people bring with them feels minuscule in the face of such an enormous idea as the space in atoms. By offering a vast imponderable image, I help the students part with their expectations, so hopefully, they can be more receptive to the present material and investigation.

Getting the teacher present

The most important person to be present is the teacher. I always direct at least some part of the warm-up to myself. During the last presidential election, my anxiety level made it difficult to lie on the floor and feel my weight—I was churning too much inside to lie still. I often would have people stand and shake and bob and do "the shivers". This would let me (and us) slough off the outside world, so we could enter a state for dancing and learning. It turns out, more often than not, what the teacher needs will be somewhat universal, or at least useful, for everyone to get into the room.

Naïve innocence

When a group gathers for the first time, the teacher gets to help shape the culture. We can model curiosity, relaxation around touch, and generosity.

When we step into a group that has been working together over time, they may have developed codes and conventions of interacting that block curiosity and learning.

One approach with a stagnant culture is to name, with naïve innocence, what is present. Sometimes, the simple act of naming a behavior can help the group move beyond it.

In Bogota, Columbia, I was invited by the Ministry of Culture to facilitate a Contact Improvisation workshop with 22 of the country's foremost dance teachers, choreographers, and dance academics.

This was one of the biggest challenges of my teaching career. These were Colombia's most accomplished in all dance forms: contemporary, folk dancing, hip hop, ballet, street dancing etc.... these were BIG personalities from decidedly diverse backgrounds. I was warned that many of this group were in direct conflict with one another.

The first day, the Ministry took two hours for introductions and then turned the floor over to me. I started by saying,

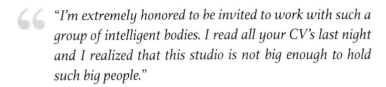

> *"I'm extremely honored to be invited to work with such a group of intelligent bodies. I read all your CV's last night and I realized that this studio is not big enough to hold such big people."*

They laughed because this is what many were thinking. I then said,

> *"The only way this is going to work is by each of us making the room bigger with our* generosity.*"*

These BIG folks then found the ground to work together by going to the side of Contact Improvisation that is about generosity. By the end of our time together, they were not only dancing beautifully, they were also holding each other with incredible care.

This is an example of, while shaking in my boots, speaking with naïve innocence.

18

HOLDING SPACE

E very day the entrance changes places
Just like with intimacy, when we dance or teach, the doorway changes places each day. One day, we get through the door by looking into each other's eyes, the next day the doorway is to be frisky, and the next day to be slow and attentive. How frustrating and how superb that we cannot rely on what we did yesterday.

N ot making sense
"Deriva" is a Portuguese word for "drifting." It's a Brazilian concept of going somewhere but not traveling in a straight line. By drifting or roaming to a destination, the journey goes from a single plane to something more three dimensional. Sometimes, teaching (and dancing) is like a child scribbling: it doesn't make sense. Don't rush these moments for yourself or your students. In the end we are not teaching techniques; we are modeling how to investigate a proposition. Scribble on.

How teachers derive their authority

While teaching at the *Seattle Festival of Alternative Dance and Improvisation (SFADI),* I had the opportunity to attend or observe classes with nineteen teachers. I gave myself the score of recognizing and articulating how each teacher derived their authority.

I identified two primary styles that I've nicknamed:

- *Alluring* authority
- *Enlivening* authority

A teacher who *allures* navigates an inner landscape; they reach into themselves and create a wake that draws their students along. An alluring teacher is more likely to give perceptual prompts, rather than tasks. They will often lay out an idea or score that is spacious – then the student becomes the piece that completes and fulfills the puzzle.

A teacher who *enlivens* projects their presence and personality to the edges of the room and creates a vessel that carries students into a new awareness or skill. An enlivening teacher often puts out complete ideas. The students discover where they stand by constellating themselves in a particular relationship to the material. An enlivening teacher is more likely to use the authority that comes from putting material into lists: "There are three kinds of falls: 1) the folding fall, 2) the rolling fall, and 3) the long fall...."

An alluring teacher is more likely to create an environment where the student finds their own variations for falling to the floor. An alluring teacher grants their students more autonomy and time for personal investigation. An enlivening teacher, on the other hand, can expediently get their students into realms and states they wouldn't have found on their own. A student flips through the air like never before when the teacher confidently leads them to this place.

I suppose a master teacher would have both styles of authority at their command, but most teachers I observed were strong in one or the other.

As a teacher who enlivens, I aspire towards (and envy) the savvy of the adept alluring teachers.

Trusting our students

How do we trust our students? One way is to imagine that each of us is a fragment – being together allows us to see a mosaic of the whole. Trusting our students helps us to see the bigger picture.

The lucid witness

While dancing, we are witnessed through the point of contact. A dance partner who is an alert witness enlivens us, deepens our sense perception; they transform us. Some of the most wonderful dance partners are those who keep the witness wide-awake to discover where we go together. The same is true with a teacher.

Give it all away

I overheard a student as she walked out of a class at the Freiburg Contact Festival exclaiming, "That teacher loves the truth so much that he hates to part with it." This reminded me to give away all I know, to not hold back.

When dancing, give the dance your full attention, your full energy, your full presence, as if this were your last dance for the entire year. The same is true when teaching. Don't withhold. Like in lovemaking, when we hold nothing in reserve and empty the bucket fully, it fills again and again.

B ridle and then unbridle the class

Pull back on the reins and hold the students in check. Offer less. Go slower than is comfortable. Then, when you loosen the reins, the students move forward on their own volition, and they need not be "spurred" on.

S taying with the material when it's uncomfortable

When we return to a single theme repeatedly with a group, it can be like digging a well. By digging in the same place, the hole gets deeper, the light of the entrance gets farther away, and it gets darker. The ground gets murky, and our hands get muddy just before we unearth water.

It helps to go into an inquiry knowing there is the potential for boredom or anxiety. By modeling tenacity, there's less chance of the group giving up just before the shovelful that unearths the artesian spring.

G etting to fast dynamic dances

One can be in a fast, whitewater dance by agitating and churning the waters. But I find it's more connected, delightful, and safe to arrive in the whitewater by beginning in the connection found in the slow subterranean rivers of sensation.

I notice adept teachers normally use this sequence from slow-connected to fast-dynamic.

B ringing vulnerability into the room

I received a valuable gift from one of my first Contact teachers, Charles Campbell. He was willing to name his feelings of vulnerability. This might be about his life or about the present moment while teaching.

The group then became willing to be present in their own vulnerability.

W hen trust is present

It is frequently on the third meeting or the third day of a workshop when people begin to trust each other enough to feel and possibly express resistance or anger. It is a healthy sign when people are willing to be in conflict with the teacher and each other. It shows we are getting comfortable and more honest together.

T he identified patient

Sometimes, a student becomes the "identified patient" of the class. People race to help him, and look to that person for the next round of angst. As a teacher, I can get frustrated by this, or I can re-direct, so this person becomes the portal through which others can find their emotional body and bring vulnerability into the room.

Often, people rush to fix this person by offering advice. As the teacher, I can redirect by saying, "Has anyone else here had a similar experience?"

Injuries

Contact Improvisation is an athletic dance form. People occasionally get injured or, more likely, reactivate old injuries.

It's a delicate moment when someone in class gets hurt. A primary feeling around injury is shame. I make sure to get attention to the person but not by the whole group. There is also the shame or feelings of guilt and responsibility of the person who was partners with the hurt person. I make sure someone checks with the partner too – "How are *you* doing?"

When a person is hurt, it affects everyone in the room. Before the end of class, I will ask the person who was hurt if they want to give an update to everyone as a way to complete the loop.

Sometimes, the incident can be reconstructed so the people involved can learn from it, and at times it can be a learning opportunity for the entire group.

It constantly amazes me how few injuries there are with the range of dynamics we bring into our dancing.

Teaching in communities with jams and with no jams

Before teaching in a new place, I find out how the jams are doing. In communities where they do little jamming, there is an appetite in workshops for dancing. In communities where there is a lot of jamming, there is a craving for exercises and material.

Working with mixed level classes

A perennial question is how to work with mixed-level classes. By working with *states* rather than skills, the skill level difference has less impact on the group. I'm regularly amazed at how Kirstie Simpson does this. She creates a state in the room, and within that state, everyone of all levels simply knows how to dance Contact Improvisation.

Working with small classes

For a class to have a self-sustaining energy, a critical mass of eight students is necessary. When classes are smaller than eight, I make it more like a private lesson, where I orient myself towards the desires of those present. I work individually, or have them pair up while some watch. I give more direct feedback and often end with bodywork.

Working with different ages

At one teacher's conference, we discussed working with different populations. Several teachers had worked with various age groups. One said, when working with children it's helpful to create an imaginary world in which they play. Have them in a field where their classmates are boulders to climb on. Put them under water and make them eels slithering along the seabed.

With the elderly, give exercises that incrementally move them past their limitations but honor each person's specific condition. "Lift your arm as far as it will go without strain. From here, take hold of your partner's arm and see if, together, without forcing, you can go higher."

With adolescents, introduce touch through specific tasks. "Touch your partner's elbow with your finger. Push their arm around until they enter a spiral."

In working with teenagers, it's important to figure out who the 'ring leaders' are and to know their names and engage and demonstrate with them.

The converse is also true; if one member seems to have a low status or is the black sheep in the group, the teacher can help integrate that person by finding and acknowledging something they are good at.

Harnessing disobedience

Inherent in the DNA of Contact Improvisation is disobedience. This form attracts rebels. How do you encourage and harness that disobedience to help you transmit the dance?

And for the students who lean towards conforming, how do you transmit a sense of rebelliousness along with the dance?

Daytime and nighttime teaching

I like to work with the Day Mind and the Night Mind when teaching. During the day, the activities lean more towards practicality, paying the bills, a specific skill. At night, there is a leaning towards metaphor, emotion, and imagination.

Three internal scores

I have three secret scores (that I'm aware of). These

unspoken scores inform my choices, the quality of the interactions, and the style of my teaching.

1. I am cultivating my students as future (or present) teachers of the form. This raises my curiosity, respect, and expectations of the people I work with. It makes me attentive to the potential for how they will inform and enlighten me in the process.
2. I am working to increase my students' capacity for inhabiting the unresolved, those times when we don't rush to plan a resolution to the moment. Like in making love, how do we hang out at the apex, without forecasting the conclusion?
3. I'm expanding their capacity for pleasure... in all its meanings.

Three secret class scores

When I teach, I'm on three trajectories:

1. Make each moment compelling.
2. Make the material cumulative, so by the end of a workshop, people are dancing like never before.
3. Teach the skills of investigating and 'labbing' with others so the research can continue for years afterwards.

What are your secret scores?

How to inspire

Sometimes, somebody says something, and it sticks to me like a burr

This happened when I heard Nancy Stark Smith talk about being a teacher of Contact Improvisation: "I don't strive to be inspiring. I strive to be 'inspire-able'."

F ollow the wildlife

If you walk on marked trails, you are likely to see other hikers. If you step onto the parallel set of trails prowled and populated by animals, you have the opportunity to observe more wildlife.

I've noticed some teachers are skilled at delving into the parallel trails, where they observe and reveal something more concealed and wild.

A score to help develop this skill: choose a place in the natural world and spend time there daily for a year. See how it changes from day to day and season to season and how you change.

I nstability in my teaching

The dance teaches us that instability leads to mobility. And great instability leads to exhilarating mobility. When a partner and I fall off-balance together, when we each give up custody of our centers, we trust the flow of the dance to take us somewhere unpremeditated.

There are many approaches to transmitting Contact Improvisation. In this quest for the unpremeditated, I like the question: Can I trust myself to accept instability in my teaching?

19

FINDING MATERIAL

C reating teaching material from dancing

There was a period when I kept observing that seasoned dancers' swinging limbs would swipe me, and there was no impact. Or someone would land on me with seemingly no weight. I became curious how these dancers were moving with no discernible mass. From this investigation, I came up with a series of exercises I call the Cotton Candy sequence. This is about filling the air with movement, moving colorfully, but also filling the *movement* with air.

We start by getting a sense of moving our arms with speed but no mass. We then close our eyes and swing an arm, and a partner puts their arm or body in the path of the swing. At the moment of contact, the swinger softens their joints, so the impact doesn't go into the partner but into the rest of their own body right down to the floor.

The next step is going into handstands while the partner gets in the way of the kicking legs. We research how one's body can take the impact when the legs are moving with intention but then encounter an unexpected obstacle.

I repeatedly notice I find material for teaching by simply noticing what I and others bring to the dance.

Ways of making contact

At one gathering of teachers, we collected words that describe ways of making contact: nuzzling, threading, knocking, grabbing, tugging, blending, signaling, mimicking, pushing, biting, inviting, pressing, sliding.

Each word is a treasure chest of teaching material.

Reverse engineer a skill into a game

Wendell Berry says, "The impeded stream is the one that sings."

One way to transmit body knowledge is to impose limitations. We learn about our other senses by being blindfolded; we discover the depth of the contact point by not letting the point roll; we detect how to express invitations through our torso when we can't use our hands to manipulate. Using restrictions, hindrances, and obstructions are wonderful ways for coming up with new material.

A skillful teaching technique and a way to create fun games is to choose a skill and to introduce its opposite; reverse engineer a skill into a game by using opposing intentions. One example is to have one member of a duet investigate the rolling point of contact in all its variations and depths. The other member of the duet investigates the dance where the contact point (by their sheer intention, rather than blocking it with their arms) *doesn't* roll.

Transmitting abilities through games brings laughter to the learning.

Peripheral vision

One of the fundamental skills we learn early in Contact Improvisation is to enter our peripheral vision, so we can fathom what is going on in the entire room. This skill leads to additional awareness, safety, and enhanced choice making.

I call this soft gaze the "whale watching gaze." When you scan the ocean for whales, you need a soft focus so unusual movement shows up. Our brains see *movement* in our *peripheral* vision.

Taking time with the skill of soft focus of the eyes becomes a soft focus of the mind and body that allows more improvisational options to appear on the horizon.

What the dance teaches about our everyday lives

When you say to a group, "Find a partner," it's fascinating to notice how people react. Some immediately make a beeline to the person they want to work with. Some look around to make eye contact. Some rock their weight back on their heels and drop their chins and eyes and wait to be chosen.

I sometimes ask people to "find a partner" and then stop the action right away and have people become aware of their default response to this task. We then try it again, but this time, I invite people to use an alternative approach to increase their repertoire.

This technique of *stopping* and *noticing* our default responses is a potent way of making the connection between what we learn by dancing Contact and what it teaches us about our everyday lives.

O ur ideal dance partner

In the same way that each of us has an inner template of an ideal mate, we carry a template for an ideal Contact dance. When we wish to enter a dance, we look through the room and, consciously or unconsciously, match people to that internal template.

A valuable exercise is to identify and articulate our ideals in the dance. This allows us to see who we might otherwise skip over because they don't fit our ideal, and possibly find new, surprisingly compatible dance partners. Identifying our template also makes it more likely to find that partner who might give us the dance our ideals seek.

Contact teachers teach their inner template to their students. Covertly or overtly, we are teaching people to be our ideal dance partners.

P utting in material, drawing out material

The first days of a workshop, I put material into the students. The last days, I draw it back out.

If I work on aerial material initially, in the later part, I will put them into dances that are spacious and welcoming of the spontaneous acrobatics of the form.

In the beginning, the material comes from me; in the end, it emerges from them.

W hen teaching on empty

(Journal entry: December 15, 2003) Tonight was my last class of the year. I have traveled to South America once and Europe twice. I have flown over 60,000 miles. Forty-two days of this year - a full six weeks - a month and a half - were spent as travel days on airplanes.

When I started teaching tonight, my voice sounded tinny. I had heard myself say these phrases a thousand times before: "Let the ground rise up to support you. Imagine yourself spreading into the floor like pancake batter."

A wave of fear surged through me. I didn't want to teach from a place of rote repetition. I had a moment of panic – are my teaching days over?

Then I got myopic, seeing what was present in that moment. We were lying on our backs. My face was tight, so I had us make faces, and then sounds, and then tighten the entire body by making fists, curling the feet back, pulling the hips right up off the floor – then releasing everything.

This led to discovering material that taught us we can un-weight any part of the body from the floor or our partner by delegating weight out to the limbs.

By allowing each moment to be the seed of the next, I again learned there is an undying reserve of originality and creativity in our present moments.

20
=====

SEQUENCING (WITH BRENTON CHENG)

E very intensive workshop had an assigned scribe to document the material at C.I.25, the 25th anniversary cele-bration of Contact Improvisation at Oberlin College.

I was fortunate to have Brenton Cheng as my scribe. Below is what he noticed, along with some of my comments about peda-gogy, the material, and sequencing.

First Day of a Workshop

H aving studied with Martin at various times over the past 3 years, I entered this project with the following associations with his teaching: tricks/games/props, juicy images, secret formulae, appeal to the spy/the trickster/the sensualist, thrives on conflict. The class begins in Wilder Dance Studio, a large, sun-lit room with a cold, hardwood floor...

As you continue with your own warm-up, I'd like you to use the image of bread dough rising and overflowing the bowl...

Most people are unmoving lumps.

Pay attention to how the body creases and folds. Notice the potential energy and power waiting at the depths of the creases...

The activity level within the class increases. The willing response of the class fills the teacher with permission to take them farther. There are sporadic moments of voicing by the students.

Allow sounds to become part of your warm-up.

The entire room erupts in vocalizing. During another 5 to 10 minutes of warming up, Martin adds occasional input.

End up lying on your side... I was just reading this morning that the reason the heart is capable of its muscular exertion during our whole lives is that built into it is a rest after each exertion.

So, I thought we'd start with a nap... imagine all the hard work is done. You decided to come. You made the time. You earned the money. You bought the airline ticket. You're here now. The work is over. Feel gravity tugging on you. Feel the floor rising up to meet you, greeting you... imagine this is all the effort you must spend during the entire class. There is nowhere you have to be. Release even the anticipation of moving.

Martin said later, often, students come in with two things that can hinder their taking in material: 1) inertia and 2) resistance. Inertia is manifested in that there is almost always some part of the body that doesn't want to move. By starting with a nap, that part is honored and feels like it, too, is welcome in class. This allows the whole person to be present.

Before class, two students had told Martin they would try to partici-pate, but jet lag and other factors might force them to leave early. This was his response. They participated in the entire class. (Resistance was dealt with later.)

5 minutes go by. Everyone is lying on their side.

Now, slowly pour onto your back and then up onto your other side. Recall the pathway you used to get there: what starts the motion, what carries it through, and what completes the motion. Now return to the other side, pouring through your back or your belly, moving as if you're not even awake.

They repeat this a few times.

As you continue to work with the floor, give it a name. Make it a real presence for you. Just name it for today.

The next time you roll up, let your legs be as straight as possible, where you can still relax.

Now, when you're on your side, find the edge of balance, that place where you're just about to fall over onto your belly or back. Spread that point wide and then, without planning it, let your body fall as one piece. Then, using the momentum of that fall, roll up onto the other side. This is the lowest "fall" we can do. Let the down become the momentum that brings you up. Let it be exhilarating. Let it be surprising.

Martin's language often has an appeal to the emotions. He has a love of "loaded" words that go beyond being anatomical/neutral. He describes his own teaching as image-based.

Notice the difference between pouring, which we did first, and falling. Pouring has qualities of fluid density and involves a control of the motion at each point. Falling is more about the momentum and about letting go.

The pouring/falling exploration is repeated from a sitting position, from kneeling, from squatting, and from standing. When this exploration is introduced, there is no hint that greater heights will be eventually explored. Martin likes to reveal his grand design as he goes, not giving away too much too early. His classes follow the model of good mystery stories.

When he demonstrates these pouring/falling pathways, he makes abundant use of his arms as landing gear but doesn't mention them. Later, he says he felt that he chose not to mention them because he was clear in his usage of them during his demonstrations.

He explains many exercises by demonstrating them, rather than describing them. He said later that he demonstrates when he wants something specific done, then the students imitate what they have seen in the demonstration, including energy level, attitude etc. When he wants the students to find their own interpretations and variations, he describes in words what he wants done or does the minimum demonstrating needed to communicate the structure of the exercise.

When we fall from a standing position, we can lead with different parts: the knees, the hips, the scalp... from this greater height, the number of pathways to the ground increases and, therefore, the number of our choices. We can fold; we can roll; we can spread, or we can do what I call the long fall, the "banana fall."

Whichever you choose, give yourself the experience of falling. As you go over, whisper the floor's name out loud, the one you gave it earlier. Whisper it affectionately.

A piece falls into place–the reason for the earlier naming of the floor. He adds this little trick of whispering the name to suspend the moment of the fall, to draw it out. They work with this material for some time.

Now, take a walk through the room. See who's here. Note what you think of each person. Who are you attracted to? Who do you want to get to know better? Who do you see and think "uh-oh"?

Now, when you meet someone else's eyes, both of you fall to the floor.

Now, when you meet eyes, put a hand on them and fall with them,

Now, two hands.

Now, two hands and lean away.

Students are now counter-balancing as they go down to the floor.

Now, two hands and lean towards.

The next time, you are up, stay up, and keep walking. Wiggle the fingers of your left hand. Your left hand is now a "magic wand". If you touch someone with your left hand, they will "crease" around your fingers to fall to the ground.

He demonstrates. When touched by the other person, he draws in at the point where the fingers touch him, almost curling his body around the hand of his partner as he spirals to the ground. The class begins walking again and working with the creasing. People are having fun with this one.

If you "crease" someone, leave your hand on them until they reach the floor.

Notice that some people, when touched, will push out from the touched area, rather than draw in and crease around it. Now, keep going, but you can use your fingers to crease someone by shooting a crease spell from across the room.

People are engaged. By vocalizing, Martin suggests adding sound effects, which everyone does.

Now, the "crease wands" are so powerful that, if you are hit, it takes you into the air before you fall.

This whole sequence of movements, starting from walking around the space, is part of Martin's "mega-workshop" in a tiny amount of time. He said later that it touches on a lot of basic skills quickly and estab-

lishes a baseline of material for the class. People can dance more comfortably together, knowing there is this common ground.

After a few minutes of the last variation (the "super crease wand"), Martin brings the energy back down and calls everyone to form a circle. This is the welcoming circle. Martin likes to have jumped right into the action before sitting down to talk. He welcomes everyone, does names, and mentions safety.

One theme I'd like to explore over the next 3 days is dancing in a bigger sphere, where the space around us becomes a tangible support for our dance... this question comes from a dance I had 2 years ago, where I started feeling the support of the space itself. Recently, I began wondering how I could teach it.

Another thing I'm interested in is how we can go into disorientation and to the edge of control and have techniques to handle it.

Next, Martin spoke of the effectiveness of one-word safety words like "No!", "Stop!", and "Back!", where inappropriate weight is coming in your direction. The group then took 10 seconds to practice shouting them altogether. This shouting session, Martin told me later, had two functions. One was to allow them to practice using the words. The other was to give them a place for their resistance to being in class or participating to play itself out. Earlier, the inertia and resistance were mentioned. Often, people have a certain resistance to being in class, which can be directed against the teacher or learning the material. This was a way to tap into that energy, to welcome it in the same way the nap welcomed their inertia.

Time for ducking practice. Get with a partner. This will be like fighting in slow-motion. One of you swings slowly at the other. The second person will duck in the direction of the swing...

He demonstrates.

If you see something coming and you just go straight down, then if it hits you, it will still have all the force of its swing. But if you duck in the direction of the swing, the force is reduced.

The class explores this in partners

The greatest challenge for the person swinging is not to show compassion at the last minute by deviating from their course, avoiding hitting the other person. For your partner to learn, you must show no mercy...

The students laugh. Martin demonstrates.

Once you get this, you can increase the complexity by swinging at a lower height, rather than speeding up...

Now, keep going, but the person ducking can allow just a little contact with the person swinging, so you follow them just a little as they go by. This is "blending".

Witnessing from the side, I see incredible, short-lived little moments of Contact dances in the middle of the swings, all with a light level of touch. Later, I suggested working more with these almost incidental point-of-contact dances. He agreed and scribbled something in his notebook.

After the class works with ducking and blending for a few minutes, he extends the motion. Demonstrating with a partner, he shows how, after the partner has swung his arm across, Martin can duck it and bring his own outside arm back, up, and over to line up with the swinging arm and roll the contact point along their backs.

The class then practices this for about 10 minutes. Martin interrupts and adds another piece, saying after the contact point has been established, the swinging person must find a pathway for the two of them into the ground.

Martin demonstrates by having his partner and himself hold flashlights. As the person swings, pointing their flashlight, the ducking person blends the beams of the two flashlights. From this agreement, it becomes easier to redirect the direction and intention of the person who swings.

I realized later that, while this last bit had little to do with the ducking and blending skill work they had just been practicing, it provided a sample pathway for integrating the skill vocabulary into a dance. Talking later with Martin, we found that, often when he teaches, movement components are placed within the context of a dance by providing pathways into or out of the movement being worked on.

Acknowledge your partner and then find a new one. We're going to work on "vacuuming".

In this exercise, one person is on all fours. The other lies perpendicular on the first person's back, with their back down. They alternate between going onto all fours and being lifted, while remaining "vacuumed" back to back. For the person on all fours moving upwards, the secret is in initiating with the eyes, and Martin goes to each group, helping the person on all fours to allow the eyes to lead the motion.

After working on this for 10-15 minutes, Martin has them return to the ducking and blending. The vacuuming exercise is a preparation for lifting using the lower back.

To the ducking and blending, Martin then adds a lift. After ducking, he uses his own outside arm, bringing it back, up, and over to hook his armpit over the shoulder of his partner, allowing him to take a ride on his partner's lower back.

(Witnessing this motion, I despair at the inadequacy of text to describe the complex physical movement.)

The class takes over a half hour to "lab" this new combination of movements. Martin goes from group to group, giving specific feedback. Several individuals need help with how to support with their lower backs. All groups are focused on the task. Most succeed by the end of the lab time.

I'd now like you to begin a dance with another by playing with dropping your head off the vertical axis, to initiate movement in and around the vicinity of another... let your eyes be free to look around... you can play with proximity to your partner... let the dance go where it will... but sometimes, you might find your head off the vertical.

They enter duets that include a lot of mid-level dancing and an ease passing through the different height levels.

Begin to look for a mutual ending.

Take two minutes to check in with your partner. Tell them your name and something unusual about yourself.

Martin ended by bringing everyone back to a circle. Each person introduced their partner by name and by an unusual characteristic. Feedback time. People mentioned enjoying the developmental approach Martin took, the moments of play, the distinction between melting (pouring) and falling. One had a desire to work more as a whole group, versus always one-on-one.

Per one student's request, we ended by lying on our backs, heads towards the center, while Martin recounted the path of material taken through the class.

Martin later said that much of the material he had introduced had come out of his explorations and teachings from the past few weeks.

He hoped to teach in an incremental way, so each person could walk away feeling they could do more than when they had first arrived. He said he believes in teaching to the most advanced person in the class, but recognized the steps leading to that level of skill must be provided.

This class had a grand design that he stuck to. Normally, he said, he prepares 3 classes ahead of time, so depending on how the class goes, he'll be prepared to take it in many directions, as needed. Here, his original plan sufficed.

L ast Words

Some themes that bridged the three days: opening the back for sensing and support, the curve of the spine and its relationship to flying, empty legs, finding support from the surrounding space. Running alongside these consistent threads were each day's topics for research: Day 1) ducking and blending, and pouring versus falling; Day 2) rolling the topside down and the bottom side up; and Day 3) moving through the backwards arch and working off-balance. Each exercise was placed into its context for dancing, either physically through movement pathways or verbally by articulating its use within a dance.

Martin tells me he feels medium-good about the 3 days. He feels like he let the material become slightly too important, and he didn't let go into greater improvisation with his teaching. Instead, he stayed more with the material he knew he wanted to communicate.

Martin's style of teaching is image-oriented, sensational, focused on dancing, provocative, and drawing from the emotions to support the physical work. There are surprise directions found in the moment and those that are quietly pre-planted. This experience of tracking the classes helped me to articulate qualities I have felt before in his classes, and for Martin, the process also served as a sometimes flattering and sometimes startling mirror of what happened in the classroom.

21

TEACHING TOOLS

T he train of self-doubt

Images can carry people's strong feelings and issues that arise in the dancing.

I find it helpful to speak about the "train of self-doubt." I offer the image of how this train often arrives on the third day. You can hear the whistle and the rhythm of the wheels on the rails as it gets closer: Chu ku ku CHU, Chu ku ku CHU, Chu ku ku CHU... accompanied by self-doubts and judgments as they come barreling down the tracks.

You might, in your own way, hear the locomotive coming, hauling freight cars with their voices of "I'm not good enough," "I'll never learn this form," "I'll probably break my neck," "Nobody, just nobody, likes to dance with me." Or: "There's no one I want to dance with," "These people are ALL insensitive!"

The image includes the notion that a train has a regularity to its passing through. By knowing its schedule, we can stand and wave as it passes; we need not get on board; we can watch until the caboose disappears around the bend.

The most common time for the train to come barreling down the tracks is when we are at the edge of what we know. It can be a good sign to hear the train because it can imply we are on the threshold of discovering something beyond the familiar.

The train image gives the student a tool to express and sort out self-doubts. A student will often say to the group something like, "Oh, the train really came through for me today," and they will state their issue in terms of the image. The issue gets spoken and heard. Then, rather than the individual, the teacher, or the group having to carry the unease, the train can bear the weight.

The train gives students a way to be heard and acknowledged. The image helps them develop a self-witness. The disclosure and vulnerability help to bond the group. Then, with an increased appreciation and trust, the group continues the investigation into the dance.

When students get queasy

Some students will get queasy or nauseous doing material that includes a lot of rolling or shifting the head below and above the pelvis. An effective remedy for the queasiness is to have people walk through the room and look at the colors of each other's eyes.

Who to demonstrate with

When demonstrating, I often work with the more skilled students, so they get a direct body transmission and won't feel like they are invariably giving something to the less experienced students. However, I also work with newcomers to the form, so the class can see the steps my partner goes through to understand what we are demonstrating.

Name games and community building

I'm fond of how name structures and introductions help to bond a group together. I sometimes have people pair up and tell each other:

- An unusual detail about yourself
- A time when you were happy
- Something you desire
- A scary experience
- The time you came closest to death
- The time you came closest to life
- A time you broke the law or a rule
- A lie you've told
- What makes you calm
- A sensual detail about yourself
- A favorite food (in detail)
- A detail about one of your parents
- Your ideal Contact class would include...

We then come back to the group and introduce our partner with their name and what we just learned about them.

(You can find over 100 name games and 'getting to know you' structures in my eBook: *Etched in Your Brain Name Games*)

Ways to find a partner

- Piece of clothing that's the same color
- Color of eyes
- Hair length

- Similar birth date
- Everyone hold out one, two, or three fingers and find someone holding out that many fingers
- Someone you haven't worked with
- Everyone stands on their knees and puts one hand up in the air. They each find someone whose hand is as high as theirs
- Find a partner with the same (or different) foot size, wrist size, or hand size

Giving roles

When I have people working in pairs, and I want each partner to take specific roles, I ask each member of the pair to choose between related images. Some examples:

- Orchid or Succulent
- Sourdough or Pumpernickel
- Jade or Opal
- Or some regional variation depending on where I'm teaching, like the Danube or Rhine rivers

Rather than say person "A" and person "B", it's more evocative to say "Amazon River, your job is to explore the rolling contact point. Nile River, your job is to explore the dance where you don't let the contact point roll."

Disruptive students

When one or a few students are being disruptive in class, you can employ the technique elementary school teachers use –

teach from the part of the room where the disruption is. Your physical presence will often cool things off.

I also find it helpful to demonstrate with the people asking for the attention.

The challenging student

I used to imagine there was a student union somewhere that sends one challenging student to each workshop. This is the one that everyone flees when you say, "Find a partner." They often end up partnering with the teacher.

When I have a difficult student, the one who is constantly leaving, who talks ALL the time in the circle, who bails on their partners, who is critical or aggressive, I find it can be calming for them to be seen. I often demonstrate with them to see what happens.

Strategies with these individuals – have people work in small groups, rather than in pairs, to dilute the experience with the person. Use ways to pick partners like "find someone with the same eye color," that is not about choice but about destiny. Sometimes, choose your partner before you tell people to find a partner, so you, as the teacher, don't *always* dance with the student union representative.

In the beginning days of this form, more people showed up who live on the edges, the folks willing to try something new. This brought in some vital people, but with them came more extreme and challenging individuals. I find that the attendance of challenging students is declining as the form becomes more mainstream.

B est time to do aerial work

There is a tendency for students to come back after a meal and hit the floor. This is when there is latent blood sugar that can be put to work. A good way to get at some effervescence is through games.

Somewhat counter-intuitively, after a meal is the best time to do aerial work.

D ealing with excess adrenaline

When a gazelle is taken down by a lion in sport and then leaves the animal alive, something fascinating happens. Shortly after the lion leaves, the gazelle will get up and "proink." It will vibrate, twitch, tremble, and jump up and down to work off the adrenaline. It then goes back to grazing.

Sometimes, after I teach adrenalizing material, like aerial work, I have the class go into proinking. We will jump up and down and tremble and shake. We are then ready to enter dancing without excess adrenaline.

T asks that deepen connection

As people are dancing, I sometimes ask them to include three tasks. One task is generally related to how we perceive time, one task is about connecting to our partner, and one task is for making the dance less precious.

These three tasks could include:

1. Find a mutual moment of stillness.

2. At some point, see your partner's eyes.
3. At some point, pinch your partner (unless they ask you to not pinch).

In the end all three tasks are about deepening connection.

Taking baby steps

I sometimes use incremental learning, where the steps are so small the students don't know how we arrive to a nuanced or acrobatic level of dancing. By arriving with baby steps, resistance need not show its face.

Then, by reviewing the class, we can retrace the steps we took to make conscious all that we have learned along the way.

Sitting in a circle

When I say let's gather and sit in a circle, there are cultural differences for where people sit. In Auckland and Berlin, people sit with a generous space between each person. Bostonians sit a little closer. In Montreal, there is almost no space between people. In Buenos Aires, they often sit touching one another.

I like to see how a group naturally arranges itself.

When making a circle, the first people placing themselves influences how the entire circle ends up. I can create a tighter or more spacious circle by calling people together and then being one of the first to sit in relationship to others.

An aesthetic eccentricity

This is a personal quirk. When I know I will be watching students work together in pairs or threes or fours, I ask them to partner with people who have a piece of clothing with a common color. For me, people working together in matching colors are aesthetically pleasing to watch.

22

STUMBLED UPON PEARLS

C ontact styles

Here's an impulsive statement: There are TWO kinds of Contact Improvisation dancers.

1. The secret rivers of sensation dancer: This dancer follows the bends and curves and nuance of sensation inside their body as their main guide.
2. The wind-in-the-face dancer: This dancer enjoys the adrenaline of being off-balance, inverted, and dancing with velocity.

We all dance with both qualities, but I've noticed almost everyone has a bias towards one or the other.

You can tell which one is your inclination because the other feels a hair too intimate. If you are a wind-in-the-face dancer, going slowly can feel overly sexual. If you are a secret river dancer, going fast can feel too intimate in its need for trust.

I'm a diehard wind-in-the-face dancer, who aspires to immerse myself in more secret rivers in my dances.

There is a third kind of Contact Improvisation dancer that I call the 'shaper of mountains'. They sculpt the space with their bodies. It's less about the movement than the design. Many of these dancers are visual learners.

I confess it's challenging to engage with the shapers of mountains in a dance. I love movement and feel that composition gets in the way. Dare I say this... I sometimes doubt they are even dancing Contact Improvisation.

The Seven Sins of a Contact Improvisation Teacher (luckily, not mortal)

1. Not speaking loudly enough for everyone to hear
2. Bemoaning about not having enough time
3. Saying, "This can't be put into language"
4. Codifying the material
5. Not accepting their own authority
6. Not taking care of their own needs and boundaries
7. Letting their own sense of inquiry die

Another sin

A teacher calling Contact Improvisation by its diminutive, "Contact Improv."

This is often what the media does when they report on the form. It's a mystery why the media consistently does this, as so few of us use this nickname.

S upporting the practice of Contact Improvisation

When people ask what they can do outside of Contact that will support their dancing, I recommend anything that will develop flexibility, strength, and release. This includes regular massage and bodywork. Part of our training and discipline is receiving bodywork!

One way to expand trust in our dance abilities is to develop overall body strength. I've regularly heard people say, "C.I. is not about strength; it's about passing your partner's weight through your bones." Passing weight through the bones is an essential ability a person brings to their dancing, but being strong brings additional colors to the improviser's palette.

When people ask, I sometimes add, anything that will develop imagination, levity, and an increased capacity for sensation and joy.

E rections

Occasionally, in or out of class, a student will bring up the question of erections while dancing. What if I get one? What if my partner gets one? At CI25, one teacher said, "Because a man can get an erection while standing at the kitchen sink washing dishes, it's best to not get too offended or too flattered if your partner has some tumescence."

If an erection is expressing a non-consensual getting off on the dance, then something needs to be changed and/or communicated. (There is much more on this topic in the essay: 101 Ways to Say No to Contact Improvisation.)

M aking room to talk about issues this dance invokes

By dancing in close physical proximity with others, we put ourselves close to issues of sexuality, violation, gender politics etc. Rather than bring up these issues, which I find can be a slippery slope, I prefer to make room for concerns to surface under their own steam, at their own time.

G ender differences

In an earlier edition of this book, I put in these two comments:

Contact Improvisation has a fairly even split gender-wise, but in most places I visit, there are more women who take leadership positions in the community. It's more likely that women will organize the festivals, set up the performances, bring in the visiting teachers, and run the jams. I wonder why.

When groups are single gender or gender balanced, they are more playful and full of beans than if there is a preponderance of one gender over another.

While these observations are generally still true, in the past decade, gender identity has become more diverse, fluid, and rich. Viewing the world through a binary lens was already complex; now there are so many hues it has become harder to make generalizations. I'm constantly reminded we have so much to learn from one another.

B ruises

People who are new to the form get bruised in obvious places, like the hip bones, knees, and elbows. More seasoned dancers get bruised in unusual places, like under the chin, or in the armpit, or on the ribs. For admission to my advanced workshops, I'm sometimes tempted to have people send in photos of their bruises :).

When I'm not at my best

One day, I taught a class that was rough around the edges because I was not feeling all that "on". A student came up to me after and hearing my lament said, "The sign of a master teacher is not how well they teach on a good day, but how they teach on a bad one."

Charismatic teachers

There is a Chinese saying about charismatic teachers: "The bigger the front, the bigger the back." I feel we have a healthy blend of respect and skepticism for charismatic leaders in our community.

Taking notes

I often tell my students: "Reviewing a class by writing it down afterwards is like getting to take the class twice – the synapses shoot off all over again. And days or years from now, when you are teaching, you will have a treasure chest from which you can adapt the material and make it your own."

The history of Contact Improvisation

Americans are swimming in the context in which this

dance was created and frequently don't care to think about the history or environment in which C.I. was birthed.

Europeans and South Americans and elsewhere are hungry for context. They are curious about the history and the ancestry from which C.I. emerged. They are more likely to buy Contact Quarterly magazine or my book of Contact essays, even if English is not their first language.

Some standard Contact courtesies and guidance

- Don't grab people's landing gear by doing things like hooking elbows when arching someone over your back. This restricts their means to take care of themselves.
- Keep your toenails trimmed, so you don't lacerate your partners.
- When on all fours with your partner's weight on your back, don't fold your toes under. If someone falls from your back to your ankles, the fall can injure your toes.
- No dangly jewelry that can hook into clothing or skin.
- Bathe regularly.

Self-consciousness around touch

I sometimes teach in dance and theater departments at universities with students who do not self-select in. They are there because it is a requirement. In these instances, I tell the story of how I started dancing at age twenty-two. When I began Contact Improvisation, I knew had found MY form, and I was committing my life to this dance.

I called my parents and said, "Mom, Dad, guess what?! I'm going to be a dancer!" There was a long silence on the other end of the phone and then they both, simultaneously, in high-pitched voices exclaimed, "Martin, NOOOO!!!"

They said, "But Martin, there's no money in it." Then they said what was really on their minds, "Martin, you're too old."

This story usually gets a laugh. I find I have the impulse to speak this story to newcomers, who might feel self-conscious with the touch. It brings lightness, levity, and some relief to the student's parental voices that might be weighing down their own shoulders.

Disaster teaching dreams

I've learned I'm not the only teacher that has these; I woke up this morning having dreamt another teaching disaster dream:

The dance studio is not available, so I must teach in the cobblestone courtyard. There are more than 100 students, and I must shout to be heard, and they still can't all hear me. No one will move to the ground – it's too hard and dirty. Some African Americans are feeling unwelcome and shut out. Wooden splinters are poking up between the stones. People keep picking them up and passing them to me as I'm teaching. I'm lugging around an armful of two-foot long splinters. No one is listening to what I'm saying...

The source of charisma

Where does charisma, that vital and ephemeral quality in a teacher, come from? Maybe it comes from the region in a person where they itch and can't reach to scratch themselves. Charisma is a way to reach out and say, "Scratch me!"

The festival teacher performance

There is nothing quite as painful for me as the festival teacher performance. Teachers, whom I love to watch dance at jams, get up on stage and suddenly lose their Contact Improvisation skills and get wildly performative by doing time/space dance improvisation and bad theater.

At the Contact Festival in Vienna, the main organizer, Sabine Parzer, introduced a different structure she calls, "Dance Bubbles". Rather than an evening performance, she put in moments throughout the festival where people could do "showings of their practice." These were simple demonstrations of the form, complete with listening and choice making and the spontaneity generated from the reflexive response to physical contact. The quality of the listening amplified by having a room filled with attentive witnesses. This structure invited people to perform Contact Improvisation.

I wish more festivals would try this format.

Dancing with beginners

More than one founder of the form has said the sign of a master dancer is not their ability to dance with other skilled Contacters, but their ability to dance with beginners. This form is not about a batch of skills dancing with a batch of skills. It's about one person meeting and dancing with another.

23

LANGUAGE

SEWING WORDS TOGETHER

L anguage is animal display

The language that flies from our mouths is animal display. Our job is to not be shy, but to encourage our language to grow hair, shed skin, and our feathered words to spread and take flight.

L anguage styles

I've identified six language styles that teachers use:

- *Task*: "Take the fingers of your right hand and reach across towards your left shoulder. Let those fingers pull you into a roll over to your belly."
- *Kinesthetic/sensational*: "Feel the distance between your hand and your torso. As you bend your arm, notice the sensation in the joints. As you allow your body to follow your hand, feel the press of your tissue into the floor as you roll over."
- *Anatomical*: "Notice how the scapula engages as the elbow flexes. Allow the metacarpal bone of your middle

finger to cross over the sternum and notice the intercostal muscles engaging sequentially down the posterior as you roll over to your anterior."

- *Imagistic*: "The floor is a huge bread board. Someone begins to tilt the board. As it tilts, you are like bread dough effortlessly pouring yourself down the incline."
- *Relational*: "Notice where you end and the floor begins. As you begin to roll, notice the different relationships created between you."
- *Play*: "When I clap, roll to your other side. If I clap twice, roll there and back. If I clap three times, roll there and back and then bleat like a sheep."

Our different voices

With almost all the language styles, I notice that both the *hypnotic* voice and the *imperative* voice are necessary for a well-rounded Contact teacher.

Using words with more impact

Sometimes, the sound of the word is more important than an accurate meaning. "What comes into your perception when you stop striving?" is more accurate, but "What comes into view when you stop striving?" has more impact.

Generating good will

When I teach a workshop where I'm entering uncharted territory, I sometimes say to my students, "Your goodwill is appreciated." This one small phrase helps get people into the investigation, rather than expecting to be fed material

Other helpful phrases· "I've never tried this before," "I'm not sure where this is going to take us, but that's what excites me."

However, when these phrases are used programmatically, they can sound banal and then the teacher can lose a vital bond with their students.

These statements show modesty in the face of what we are researching. If a teacher habitually makes themselves small, it is best not to use these phrases.

A wakening the psyche when you have something important to say

At my first men's conference with Robert Bly, he said, "I'm going to describe the seven male modes of feeling." At the next conference, he said, "Here are the three male modes of feeling," and at the next, "thirteen male modes of feeling." I asked him at dinner, "What are you up to?" He laughed and said, "When you give a list, people's psyches run for pen and paper. It wakes people up."

We so desire order in our lives that the promise of a list gets our attention. The truth is, there is no fixed number. When I say in class there are three ways to fall to the floor, people look up expectantly, and some actually reach for their notebooks. By constantly changing the number, two purposes get served: you wake people's attention, and the students AND teacher learn not to be controlled by the tyranny of lists.

It's not true to say there's only one rule in Contact Improvisation. But saying "there is only one rule" makes people alert to what you are about to say.

At the beginning of every workshop, I say a variation of this: "There is only one rule in C.I. and that one rule is – take responsibility for yourself. Your partner can't be in your body. I, as the teacher, can't be in your body, so it's important that *you* be in your body. Please keep a part of you awake, able to communicate, physically or verbally, what you need and desire."

Another way I'll introduce this is to say, "There is one muscle that is more important to have strengthened in Contact Improvisation than any other muscle. That is the muscle of self-responsibility...."

By saying "one rule" and "more important," I'm alerting people they to be awake for what they are about to hear.

Giving images to contain strong feelings

Some teaching material can take people over a physical or emotional edge. This material might stir up fear or other strong feelings. Imagery can be invoked, so these emotions can support, rather than hinder, the investigation.

I have a leader/follower exercise, where the follower moves with their eyes closed. This gets dynamic with the follower running through the room with no touch by the leader. It is scary to keep running and to trust that your partner will redirect you or stop you before you hit the wall.

I offer the image that the person is on a safari being led by a guide. They are taken to see lions and gazelles; they go spelunking and bungee jumping. Inherent in the imagery is danger, so the fear can be placed in the image and the person can loosen up within the fear. (I also invite people to shout and vocalize.)

Right after both my parents died, it was hard to dance because the vulnerability of dancing took me into my bereavement, and tears would flow down my face. Then I came up with the image, "bones softened by grief." When I would dance (and teach), I would invoke this image. The grief could then allow a softening in me that supported the dancing and my engaging with people.

(For more on this, see "The train of self-doubt" in the chapter, Teaching Tools).

Teaching an art form

I've noticed, when teachers talk about the "discipline" of our practice and speak about "research" and "investigation," it wakes the students up to engage in this dance as an art form, rather than Contact being simply recreational and an act of pleasure seeking.

Defining the words we use

It is irresponsible to use big words without defining them first. Before we use words like *release, energy, allow, consciousness*, it is our task as teachers to do the labor of definition.

Certain words have been so overused they are dead fish and should almost never be spoken, except ironically. These include: *transformation, share, journey, amazing, quantum, deep,* and any combination of words that use: *paradigm.*

"Go deep into your experience," has no meaning. A teacher must ask, "What do I mean by 'deep'?" and then do the work to define it.

When a teacher has the discipline to work with language, they bring more clarity to their teaching. They also teach with more poise and command more authority.

Apology words

If I'm tired or not in top form, I'll use more "apology" words and phrases. Some examples of these are when I say, "We are going to take *just* another minute." "*Please* come to this side of the room." "Take a *really* deep breath." "Now *I would like you* to move near the edges of the room." These apology words are extraneous — they hurt the communication or transmission of the material or the form. I mostly forgive myself for using them.

Opening a circle to talk about their experiences

When we circle up to speak our experience, how do I, as the teacher, open the floor so people can speak to all sides of their experience? I often combine, "What were your discoveries?" and "What were your challenges?"

Ray Chung simply asks: "What did you observe?"

Priming the discussion

Here is a technique used by several teachers to prime a class for discussion. Everyone takes a slip of paper and writes on it this sentence completion: "In Contact Improvisation, I'm afraid of..." or "In Contact Improvisation, I don't like..." or "In Contact Improvisation, I struggle with..."

The slips of paper are folded and thrown in a pile. Everyone takes one out and reads it as if it were their own. Some are funny, some are poignant, some are painfully truthful. After the statements are read, the floor is opened for whomever would like to speak.

Tools for generating discussion and reflection

- Posit a question at the beginning of class and come back to it at the end. This becomes the research question.
- Go around the circle and everyone throws in a word or a phrase, then open the discussion.
- Have people talk in pairs. I then say, "Finish this sentence and let's continue as a group."
- Have people recall moments from the class or the dances.
- Go around and everyone asks a question before opening the discussion.

Giving questions rather than findings

How do you generate an investigation in people by offering a question, rather than your finding?

Here is a question: There are a few teachers who have the capacity to create an environment where the learning feels sacred – where rules and regulations are replaced by art and beauty – where Eros replaces morality. How do they do that?

Some phrases I find helpful

- Dance a hair less with your ideal and a hair more with your partner.
- Suspend your disbelief you will ever warmup.
- Don't rush the awkward moments.
- Don't drown/wallow in the sensation.
- Dance with the body you have now.

- Don't rush a sense of connection.
- We are building our comfort for the awkward, we are building our capacity for the unresolved.
- Let gravity do its job.
- Leading is 90% listening.
- Great instability leads to great mobility.
- Become more involved *with* and less dependent *on* your partner.
- The work we are doing today makes us part of evolution of the form.
- Let this moment be the seed of the next.
- Let this movement be the seed of the next.
- A seasoned dance partner has several relatable places at a time.
- If you find yourself 'efforting' or 'working' or if you get distracted, pause. Pause to replenish your curiosity.
- Lifts: make it a film, not a photo.
- If at first you don't succeed, try less.
- What is the smallest stretch you can still feel?
- Dance with this question: What is too little tone?
- What am I not perceiving? What is at the edge of my perception?
- What is obvious right away and what gets revealed with time?

24

GIVING FEEDBACK

The luminous kick in the pants

Some teachers are skillful at holding space for people to change and evolve at their own pace. Some teachers are adept at providing a luminous kick in the pants. I aspire to provide both.

Why give feedback?

Nancy Stark Smith has challenged my beliefs about Contact Improvisation more than once. When she and I co-facilitated our first CITE (Contact Improvisation Teacher's Exchange) at Earthdance, I offered a structure to practice different methods for giving feedback to students. Nancy challenged me to articulate WHY we, as teachers, give feedback. To what end? She asked, "Are we simply trying to transmit our aesthetic onto someone else?"

Fortunately, CITE was a few months away, so I had time to mull these questions.

I realized I have two intentions in giving feedback.

The first is safety. I give cautionary pointers when I see dancing where there is potential for the dancer, their partner, or someone else in the studio to get hurt. These tips often include specific details like, "stay aware of everyone in the room," or "refrain from grabbing your partner's landing gear," or "don't hook and yank." If I see a wild dance that has a perilous level of unconsciousness, I will join the dance or interrupt the dance and directly say something like, "Your dancing is scaring me. Please be more aware of the room."

The other feedback is what I give to a student or a dance partner. My motive in this feedback is to open additional worlds in people's dancing. When I watch or dance with a student, I might sense an ability they are on the threshold of discovering. Or I might sense something whose embodiment would help round out their dancing. To give feedback, I look through the lens of this question: "What worlds are waiting to open up?"

In giving feedback to a student, my perspective is limited; I'm human after all. This is why I recommend that students study with many teachers. This way, they get many reflections from many viewpoints. I know that, after dancing and teaching for almost 40 years, my perspective is not insubstantial. I can often offer a recommendation that will have a person dancing like they've never danced before. There is satisfaction in this for both of us.

A structure to learn how to give feedback

Here is the feedback styles structure I offered at CITE and at teacher's conferences on four continents.

In groups of six, there are three (or more) rounds where a duet is witnessed by four people. Each of the four witnesses chooses a feedback style beforehand and gives feedback in that style after the dance. The dancers have a non-performative dance as if they were at a jam lasting about ten minutes.

The feedback styles include;

More general feedback:

- Simply report what you saw (not what you liked/disliked)
- What you liked seeing and would have liked to see (rather than what you disliked)
- Giving an Image to dance with (More on this in the next chapter)

More specific feedback:

- Welcome an awareness: "Notice where your head is in space when your feet leave the floor."
- Hands on feedback – trace the pattern, show the option
- Using their eyes. Have them repeat a specific movement: "Watch my hand."
- A question: "What if, when your feet leave the floor, you can see behind yourself?"
- Demonstrate the habit and the alternative(s)

We do several rounds of dances, so each person gets to practice several kinds of feedback and gets to receive diverse feedback in different styles from different viewpoints.

Feedback structure for mixed level groups

Here is a variation on the feedback structure for mixed level groups. I call it "By Request Feedback."

Each dancer names what they are currently interested in with the dance. They articulate the area where they would like feedback based on their current research. This way, the witnesses look with the lens the dancer has requested.

I normally give examples to prime the pump. Your lens might include:

- How are the qualities of my dancing different when I have my own center and when I give my center over to something mutual?
- When do I bail on lifts and rides?
- How do I dance differently with men and women?
- What are the moments when I retreat from the follow through and turn back?

F inding what kind of feedback is useful

Feedback can lead to questions. The questions can be a guide to the kind of feedback a person is more receptive to.

W hen a person seems stuck

I sometimes run across students who, over time, appear to fear spontaneity or who are unwilling to take risks; there is no outward sign of movement or growth or change.

I now recognize I'm obliged to make a subtle distinction here. There are those who are resistant and need encouragement and prodding, the luminous kick in the pants. On the other side, there are those who are in chrysalis, something embryonic in them is forming, and they need spaciousness for their change to occur.

For those in stasis, something profound is taking place, but hidden from view. In these cases, it's important NOT to push – to let the person evolve at their own pace – into their own form.

I have struggled with how to recognize the difference between the state of resistance and the state of metamorphosis. I wish the signs were easy to recognize outwardly. The only hint I can give is that it becomes clearer when you touch the person. Someone in resistance has a knee-jerk defiant "no" in their tissue. Someone in metamorphosis has a core that feels fluid and in motion, a feeling of all-embracing vulnerability.

Giving memory cues

Most people who dance Contact Improvisation are kinesthetic learners. When giving feedback about something that happened during a dance, it's helpful to let the person know where they were in the room when it happened. This gives a memory cue, which is especially helpful to kinesthetic learners, to help the person remember what they were doing in that moment.

Giving feedback during jams

When I'm dancing with someone at a jam, I rarely give comments on their dancing. However, some people long for reflection as part of their investigation. If I notice something that might be useful for my partner, I'll ask if they are open to hearing it. It's handy to receive information during a dance because the dance can continue and the feedback put right to use.

Framing feedback to the local culture

In different cultures, they give distinct kinds of feedback. After a class in the USA, students are likely to come up and say something like: "Great class, you sequence material well. I would have liked more falling material."

In Europe, especially central and northern Europe, where they are more reserved about praise, on the fourth day of an intensive, I might hear something like, "I enjoyed the imagery," or "I have no regrets coming to your workshop."

In South America, it's not uncommon for a student to take me by my arms and say, "You changed my life!"

The local style of giving feedback can be a guide to how a teacher frames their feedback to the students.

Giving written feedback

When people receive feedback, it can touch a nerve, and the person might get defensive or emotional. I find, mostly, when being direct, it's best to be direct. If I hedge, it will be felt.

I've also noticed that written feedback is easier to receive. Before, where I might lean in and whisper something to people dancing, I now have written statements I hold up for a person to read. I also keep empty cards, so I can write things down in the moment to show the person. I call this "feedback on the fly."

Here are some statements I might show a dancer:

- Relinquish your center
- Enter spirals
- Follow through

- Drape
- Your ribs are fingers
- You have fish eyes
- Be safer
- Take the energy in your eyes and put it in the contact point
- Take a hair longer with everything
- 90% listening
- A hair less precious
- Feet like schools of fish
- Read the floor through your partner
- Be pushy
- Follow aggressively
- Get what you want
- Narrow base
- Where is everybody?
- Remember
- Leave something behind

Having a comment that's written somehow bypasses the self-judgement area. I've found this to be true across cultures.

25

TO THE HEART OF FEEDBACK

GIVING IMAGES

Once I have pointers to give, the question becomes how to give them. What is the most accessible and utilizable way to transmit observations? Do I give a specific tool or task? Do I make them aware of some well-worn pattern blocking other possibilities? Do I give a question, or demonstration, or give feedback through my hands?

Over the decades, I've found the most effective feedback to introduce new worlds into people's dancing comes in the form of an image. I translate my observation into an image for the person to invoke while dancing.

If I dance with someone and they have a collapsed demeanor, I might ask them to notice when the dance becomes rambunctious and to imagine they have a mane of a lion whipping in the wind. How does this affect their movement, their ability to organize, to support, to cartwheel, to fill space, to be strong?

A situation I regularly see is a person going into their backspace to receive support on their partner. As the dancer lays back, their chin habitually tucks, leaving their head with a vertical orientation to the room around them. This tucking stiffens the neck and spine, reducing their ability to listen and respond to the abundance of pathways available.

There are several kinds of feedback I can give here. I can describe what I'm seeing and give the tool of looking for the floor behind them. With touch, I can guide them, so their head follows the spine and goes backwards. I can have them visually watch my hand as they go back, so they must drop their head to keep my hand in their visual frame.

While each of these is useful and each has its place, the correction is specific and local. My preference is to suggest to a person they invoke this image while dancing: "You have the eyes of a fish, and you can see the full 360-degree sphere around yourself." Not only can this image lead to the head and upper back opening into the backspace, but the orientation of their dancing, in general, can become more spherical and multi-directional.

This is not a local fix. Images can take longer, but they work systemically.

The more striking an image, the more useful it is. "Your blood is heated" is okay, but "You have jalapeño peppers in your blood" is better at getting to the entire circulatory system of someone's dance. It is valuable to give physical corrections and to offer specific techniques, but I have found that imagery is what brings down mountains and sets the oceans ablaze.

How do I come up with the images? I often set up structures where people are dancing, and I move around the studio and witness as if my body was a dowsing rod. I witness viscerally. I notice when my body is drawn in and when it falls back on my heels. From this place, I ask the question, "What worlds are waiting to open up?"

Often an image appears. Over the years, I've found that, some-

times, the image is directed towards a person's dance and, sometimes, towards their personality. These two are so intertwined I
often can't tell the difference. In our dancing or in our lives, what
threshold is about to open?

I can use an image to ground someone more in sensation. I
might say, "You have pads of butter between each vertebra,"
or "You have a perfectly ripe pear dangling in your solar plexus,"
or "Cat whiskers all up and down your spine."

If I see a person putting in so many ideas and impulses they
crush what the dance is offering, I'll give an image like: "Kissing
for miles and miles," or "You have mermaid's hair floating
behind you."

To get someone to improvise from a more visceral place, I might
offer, "Your dance radiates out from your ovaries," or "You have a
prehensile tail.""

Some images challenge people's self-view and are aspirational.
"Drop your reins and let your animal carry you," or "You are
sleeping beauty right after the kiss." (What if I *have* been asleep
for one hundred years?)

I try to stay aware when an image is not sinking in. If visual
images don't seem to work, I'll try an acoustic image like: "You are
the vowels of the alphabet," or "Tuning all the strings of the
violin."

I need at least six days with a group to have an image ready for
everyone in a workshop. The longer I work with a person, the
more I have them in my visual field, have felt their body indelibly
imprinted on mine by dancing together, the more likely I am to
find a helpful and accessible image. Once I know the images are

ripe, I'll have everyone sit together to hear each other's feedback. This allows people to recognize how personal each image is to the individual and how it stands in contrast to the others.

Sometimes, I flesh out an image with a story or other accompanying images. I ask people to resist the temptation of trying to interpret the image or to figure out my intention in giving it. The treasure in the image comes by noticing what's stimulated by evoking it while dancing. The image is more powerful than our interpretation. The aim is to summon the image with curiosity and openness. When I give the image to a woman, "You are a man," they are not to pantomime flexing their muscles and strutting around bow-legged. Just by invoking the image, they will have a physical response. It's saying the phrase to yourself, "I am a man," and allowing what comes up to influence the dance.

After everyone in the circle receives their image, we return to dancing. At any moment until the end of the workshop, anyone can offer a bird call to the room. As we dance, if we hear a 'cheep', we take that as a prompt to invoke our image. This way, people can get in the habit of invoking their image to see what changes.

It puts a skip in my step when I receive emails from people after years or even decades thanking me for all they received from their image.

Gallery of Images

In old fairytales, you sometimes find a character who bears gifts. In one Grimm's tale, *The Spirit in the Bottle,* his name is Mercurius, one name of Hermes, the god of boundaries and transitions. These gifts might include a bottle of wine that never empties, a cane to knock on any door and the door will open, or a cloth that will heal any wound or illness.

Here is a pocket-sized gallery of some images I use in my dancing and my teaching. I rarely categorize them because many would fit under several headings. However, to show you how they can be useful for giving feedback, I've categorized them here.

Letting Go of Tension

- you are your childhood rag doll
- jellyfish in the joints
- patina cracking and peeling off
- spaghetti as it's dropped into boiling water
- the earth is breathing you

Increasing Capacity for Sensation

- your ribs are fingers
- your home is in your partner's marrow
- your tongue weighs ten pounds
- slightly sunburned all over your body
- your marrow speaks: hear
- the ale after the froth has settled

Letting Go of the Head

- you have a mink curled up in your skull
- itchy, sunburnt skin on your upper back
- eyes that see 360 degrees all the time
- mermaid's hair floating behind you
- you have a prehensile tail coming out of the top of your head

Sensitivity

- you're a pickpocket
- the weight of your shadow
- the pelvis is a tongue tasting the dance
- all your body parts are labia
- your partner is slightly sunburnt
- your family has been dancing for three generations: your partner's family has been dancing for four generations – what can you learn from them?

Increasing Ease

- 100 hands are doing it for you
- pads of butter between each vertebra
- spine is a string of pearls
- you are the vowels of the alphabet
- slippery soap bubbles in all your joints
- you are the Amazon river

Ease with the Floor

- bread dough rising and overflowing the bowl
- sausages for bones
- the floor is the belly of a giant
- pancake batter spreading as it's poured
- gravity comes from all around you and holds your skin on
- you have a tail (prehensile or not)

Giving Support

- granite mountain with crags and ledges and trees growing from crevices in the rock

- you are a philanthropist
- you are the nose of a circus seal
- your throne is in your pelvic girdle

Body Awareness

- fingers/toes are sparklers
- tongues between each vertebra
- tongues in your hip folds
- a perfectly ripe pear dangling in your solar plexus
- cat whiskers all up and down your spine
- a heart-shaped pendant that glows hanging from your sternum (or sacrum or shoulder blades)
- pendant with a precious stone of your choosing hanging from your perineum
- breath through your gills

Levity

- helium balloon in the pelvis
- you are pollen
- the cloak of invisibility
- bones so porous you breathe through them
- bird bones that are lighter than feathers
- the dolphin's smile
- bones give off effervescence

Filling Yourself: Filling the Dance

- hunter after big game, deep in the jungle, and the lions have just come into view
- you are a femme fatale
- you are a Picasso painting
- the dance is illicit

- you are a seven-foot-tall basketball player
- pick up the reins and confidently lead your horse
- your body is a jungle
- mane of a lion whipping in the wind
- dance as if you're a Shakespearean actor

Inviting the Unknown

- heart is drunk
- joints are drunk
- blood is carbonated, champagne, effervescent
- drop your reins and let your animal carry you
- resonating chambers in the body – and on the chamber walls are prehistoric paintings

Letting Go

- you're molting
- just after the lovemaking that brought you to tears (the good tears)
- a teaspoon of molten gold in your solar plexus
- you just finished great lovemaking – your lover has run you a bubble bath, filled it with flower petals, put on music and lit candles. Your image is the moment of lowering yourself into this bath

Confidence

- blind woman's trust for her dog
- you fluently speak seven languages
- think of yourself as a timeless piece of literature
- your family has been doing this for 3 generations; it's not personal (or it's deeply personal)
- golden light of the moon reflecting off your chest

- dance radiates out from your ovaries

Find Energy

- jalapeño peppers in the blood
- the spider bite that makes you dance
- when the yeast realizes there is sugar nearby
- plumage like a peacock
- tuning all the strings of the violin
- you are the froth on the ale
- one shot of tequila
- a wolf howling at the moon

Healing

- greenhouse for winter blossoms in the chest
- flowing skirt, looonnnggggg hair, dangling earrings, dozen bracelets, emerald in bellybutton, tattoo of a rose on the thigh
- you're a man (for women)
- you're a woman (for men)
- in god's hands
- bones softened by grief
- you are the bride: radiating

Connection

- kissing for miles and miles
- what springtime does to the cherry trees
- a lover's hand feeding you

The Sublime Dance

- a single drop in a still pond
- the reverence, standing in a grand cathedral with sunlight streaming in
- the reflection on a lake on a windless day
- the sand spilling through an hourglass
- the sound of winter
- the quiet thread at the center of great art
- sleeping beauty after the kiss

26

NUTS AND BOLTS

TOURING CONTACT ARTISTS

C rowd sourcing the dance

In the world of computers, there is a revolution happening, called open source programming or crowd sourcing. An app is written, and then anybody who wants to can improve the source code. Linux and Mozilla's Firefox are well-known crowd-sourced apps. Creating software nobody owns that has no central control that anybody can try to improve creates apps that are the most useful, bug free, and elegant.

Contact Improvisation is an open source dance form. Everyone who enters this dance adds their discoveries and innovations. And like open source software, there is no central control. There are means of communication, so people keep track of what is going on in the network. We have the Contact Quarterly magazine, numerous Facebook pages, teacher's gatherings, and the simple fact that, when we dance, information moves between us.

This is not Balanchine or Graham technique, or Microsoft corporation, where information is imposed from the top down. Contact Improvisation is a constellation of dancers, each informing the others. Contact is an inherently unfinished dance form: Each person gets to complete it with themselves in each moment. This is the strength of the form and why it keeps fanning out worldwide.

I hope C.I. never becomes trendy, because trendy things usually end. I don't see that happening because our dance doesn't have flash; it's not out trying to colonize the world. What we have is an international group of committed practitioners, each contributing their piece to the dance puzzle. As the dance enlightens us, we enlighten the form.

Teachers are a vital part of the open source. We are one of the means of communication as we conduct the threads of what is being investigated from one part of the world to another.

Contact nomads

There is a rare breed of dancers I call the Contact Nomads. These are dancers of no fixed address. They travel across the globe from Contact event to Contact event, dancing, teaching, and performing. They are important to developing our form, as are all the touring Contact artists. They dip into the flowers of the Contact communities and then pollinate from one to another.

Working with a translator

When teaching with a translator, it's preferable to have someone not taking the class. When the translator is participating in an exercise and gets involved in their sensation, they can lose track of their role or even lose the ability to engage with speech.

Before class begins each day, I meet with the translator to go over any challenging concepts, words, or images, so they don't get blindsided by how persnickety I am with language.

Some particularly challenging concepts to translate from English are "draping" and "follow through."

I invite my translator to match me energetically. I give them examples of my 'hypnotic voice' and my 'imperative voice' so the same tone and dynamic comes across in the translation.

I find it's an intimate relationship with someone translating my words. They become my voice. I often fall in love with my translators.

Dealing with jet lag

Jet lag makes me off-kilter and discombobulated. This can lead to a dip in my self-confidence (especially on the third day). I was once given practical advice for teaching overseas: Take sleeping pills on the flight over and for the first couple of nights there. A good rest on the flight helps make the transition smoother.

Some natural options include: melatonin, valerian and a lavender bath.

Regional dance dialects

I used to differentiate the Contact styles in different parts of the world. Two decades ago, if you sat at a jam on the West Coast in the USA or in South America and squinted your eyes, you would see more weight exchange, more time off-balance, more risk-taking and spontaneous acrobatics. You would also be more likely to see people having an angry dance, or a sexual dance, or a tearful dance.

If you squinted your eyes on the East Coast, the dancers had more of their solo in place, and they would keep their centers more autonomous. If you squinted your eyes at a jam in Europe, the dancers often left physical contact to enter their solos with strong developed idiosyncrasies.

Now I feel the styles have cross-pollinated and become more mixed. While these generalizations are still true, they are becoming increasingly subtle.

I used to talk about regional "Contact styles." But people would often put a value judgment on one style over another (including me). Now I prefer to speak of "regional Contact dialects."

Cultural preconceptions

When I'm preparing to go to a country for the first time, I attempt to excavate my preconceptions and prejudices about that culture.

When I first went to Russia, I had a lot of childhood voices about the Russians being the enemy. One thing I heard several times was, "The Moscow subways are dazzling, filled with chandeliers, and beautiful mosaics to show off. But they don't care about their people; they don't even have benches for people to sit on."

When I brought this up in Russia, they said, "Why would you need benches when there are trains every two minutes?"

Cultural styles

There are different cultural styles of talking when we gather in a circle to speak of our experiences. In North America, someone will most often talk the moment the last person finishes speaking. In central Europe, people wait about three beats before talking. In Finland, they wait a full eight to twelve beats before the next person speaks (I'm glad I was alerted to this beforehand). In South America, it's not unusual for people to work up to talking simultaneously.

N oticing the culture's way of giving feedback

I attended my first ECITE (European Contact Improvisation Teacher's Exchange) in Copenhagen in 1994. I had a wonderful dance with a Danish woman, and later, I was standing with her and a few others in conversation. At one point, I said to her, "Thanks for our dance. I'm impressed by your physical intelligence and all the surprise pathways we found." After I said this, she backed into the wall as if I had punched her.

Later, when we talked, just the two of us, I asked her what had happened in that moment. She said, "Here (in the Nordic countries), we don't like to be raised above each other because then people will cut you down. We don't compliment one another, especially in public." At this ECITE, I realized my feedback would have to be sensitive to cultural differences.

C ontact Improvisation and money

The tuition for a workshop in massage, yoga, or any therapeutic skills costs substantially more than a workshop in Contact Improvisation. The pay for a C.I. teacher is consistently lower than in these other fields. I know several talented C.I. teachers who didn't continue in the field because there is "no money in it." It's a shame.

Some teachers have such an issue around money they don't even bring up the topic when invited somewhere to teach. I feel it does us all a disservice when teachers are not clear about what they are worth and what they charge. It became evident that I needed to be crystal clear about what I was earning as I returned home to a family of six mouths to feed.

P aid to travel

There was one year I spent 42 days on airplanes traveling to and between workshops. This translates as a full six weeks, a month-and-a-half spent traveling. I realized I needed compensation for that time spent hurtling through space in a cramped seat in a narrow cylindrical tube. Now I ask for a travel stipend for every city I visit, so I receive at least a token amount for my travel time.

Part of this travel stipend gets donated to environmental causes.

M y touring conditions

Many C.I. teachers simply ask for 100 Euros an hour to teach. I do it a little differently. When I'm invited to teach, I send a letter with my workshop descriptions, my bio, and my touring conditions. Below is the part of the letter I send out with my requirements:

> *When I travel to teach, every situation is different as are the financial arrangements. Sometimes I'm at schools, sometimes in private workshops, and sometimes at festivals. Below is normally what people pay me for traveling to their hometowns (and countries) and teaching:*

For workshops (All in Euros):

* 1/2 *teaching day: 3 hours: 300 a day minimum or* 45%** *of the gross revenues, whichever is greater.*

* *Full teaching day: 6-7 hours: 425 a day minimum or* 45% *of the gross revenues, whichever is greater.*

* *Travel expenses (in advance). I'm tall, so on long flights over the ocean, I fly premium economy or in an exit row.*

* *Plus a one-time stipend per city for my travel time of* 145 *(a portion of this goes to carbon offset my travels)*

* *The hospitality my hosts offer comes in many forms. People generally put me up in their homes and feed me, or I'm put up in an apartment with a per diem. I like to sleep in a real bed in a room with a door that closes.*

* *Occasionally, I like to invite one of my protégées or a friend as a guest. And often my hosts invite a helper or two as their guests.*

* *A nice dance studio, preferably with a wood floor.*

Full-day workshops normally go for six and a half, like from 11-5:30 with a break for a potluck, where people bring light food to share. This is good for community building.

We can talk about these details to see what works for all of us.

** Percentage of the gross revenues goes up to 55% or 60% if there are no travel costs involved.

The minimum goes up substantially if I'm teaching in an institution, where the percentage of the gross is not considered.

Sometimes I earn only my minimum, though this is rare. This gets balanced out when I have a full workshop, say 30 to 40 students, where I can earn over a thousand Euros a day. When I earn well, I'm pleased that my hosts also earn well for their efforts.

Teaching at festivals

Festivals are amazing beasts. There is great nourishment in rubbing shoulders with other teachers and their research. I get to connect with many new students, and festivals are a source for future workshop invitations.

However, I struggle with how little festivals typically pay their teachers. I always ask up front for a hundred euros an hour when I'm invited to a festival, but I rarely get it. The lack of income means I can only afford to attend one festival a year.

When Contact festivals first came into being, I proposed to the organizers to have me at the festival and to add an intensive workshop, before or after. This allowed me to have the nourishment of the festival and the paycheck of the intensive workshop combined. The organizers had to only pay the airfare once. This is now a common practice to bring "big name" teachers to festivals.

Teaching at home

When I lived in the Berkeley, Bay Area, I was one of the few teachers who regularly had full classes. I liked to run two simultaneous 3-month series of 12 classes each. This gave me the satisfaction of working with a committed group over a long period and meant I only needed to fill my classes about three times a year.

Like many teachers, I'm not fond of the foraging needed to get students to sign up for my classes. So, I came up with a formula to make the work palatable. I called it Hours Plus One.

When it came time to gather students, I would add up my teaching hours: 48 hours and add one hour: 48+1=49 hours. This would be the number of hours I would spend promoting my workshops.

I split my pay between my teaching hours and my promotion hours, so I was earning a substantial amount an hour for both. This made letting people know about how much they would enjoy the workshops less onerous. It also allowed me to "pay" myself to go to jams because this was part of the foraging.

When my classes started doing well, I added a prerequisite to attend. People needed to study with someone else to join my classes. This helped other teachers, and it filled my classes with students committed to the form, who were dancing several times a week.

The sliding scale

People attracted to Contact Improvisation sometimes live on a delicate edge, financially. Many in our community put little attention on material gain. This brings up how to make workshops accessible to all, while generating enough income to pay the teacher a living wage.

In the past, I've disliked sliding scales because I find they generate shame in people who pay at the low end and resentment in the people who pay at the high end. I find this affects the feelings in the studio and people's receptivity to the material.

Then Todd Paulsmeyer came up with the sliding scale, included below, for the Moab Jam. By being this specific about who is who and doing it lightheartedly, there is little residual challenging feelings around the money. Earthdance and many workshop hosts now use a variation of this system for defining their sliding scales.

I recommend a large spread between the top and bottom tuition amounts, so it becomes possible for individuals with genuine low-income situations to participate.

Student Rate:
Economically deprived students and the unemployed: $____

Regular Rate:
Employed but economically challenged (teacher, librarian, lots of kids etc.): $____

Professional Rate:
Actually contributing to your retirement plan (support the arts!): $____

O n being a freelance touring dance artist
    I saw this posted in the window of the Chamber of Commerce in Berkeley, California: "The best thing about being self-employed is you only have to work half days, and you get to choose which 12 hours."

G oing on tour with a score
    When I leave on tour, I sometimes ask my wife, Liza,

"What's my score?" One time, she replied: "Your score is wild receptivity." I asked this question to Anado, a man in my men's group, and he said, "You are so happy when you return from tours, and you've discovered new material, so your score is: make shit up." My friend Sky, who knows me well, replied, "Do what you do so well and slow down the arc of time."

So that year, my scores during my tours were: wild receptivity, make shit up, and slow down the arc of time.

Supporting the local Contact community: jam building

I often hear a lament in communities that there aren't enough people to maintain a jam. In these cases, I recommend getting together a smaller group to lab the form. Then, when there are a few committed folks, I give the following format to create a thriving jam.

I live on an island of only ten thousand people, and we have two well-attended weekly jams. We found the secret is to have multiple hosts who rotate holding the space. Each gets to host in their own way: Some choose to open the space; others like to lead warmups and hold opening and closing circles; we each get to follow our interests. The host makes sure newcomers feel welcome, though all the hosts present share in this responsibility.

Each host is responsible about once a month. At least five hosts will be present at each jam. This means people never have to question whether there will be a critical mass. We average 15-20 participants.

We keep the price of the jam low, so money is not an obstacle. The hosts also pay to attend. We've agreed that, at the end of the year, if there is a shortfall, we split it (this has never happened), and when there is a surplus, we treat ourselves to a dinner together.

I offer this formula to communities, knowing full well that thriving jams means more touring teachers will be invited to teach and pollinate the community.

Having a life beyond teaching

When I'm on the road teaching, I'm in my niche. I thrive. I get to see foreign cultures and communities as a guest, rather than as a tourist. I'm fed the local cuisine, given a bed, and presented with a group with whom I can present, and be appreciated for my love of Contact Improvisation. It makes me glow.

When I come home from my tours and, once again, I'm changing diapers and telling our fourteen-year-old that *yes*, it is *his* turn to empty the dishwasher... and then need to run through the house to find out who moved the plunger... and discover the car must go the mechanic because, when you turn the key, it sounds like someone is trying to squeeze a cat into a blender – the realities of home and family life can quickly remove the glow from being the 'celebrated' Contact teacher.

The other side of this (there seems to be always another side...) is the emptiness of the never-ending travel and countless fleeting relationships. And there is a fullness that can only come from baby shit under the fingernails, because your baby laughs when you make faces and bounce up and down buzzing like a bumblebee.

Nothing left unsaid

When I leave on tour, something dies in me.

I make sure nothing is left unspoken when I go (just in case). And then I mostly have extraordinary experiences on the road: The connections, the dances, the rubbing shoulders with different people changes me.

On my last tour, I was dancing in Uruguay, and this phrase came to me: "My life for a dance!"

27

EMBERS IN THE HEART

TEACHER'S SECRET SCORES, TOOLS AND SPICES

The teacher as alchemist

I teach in a converted colonial convent completed in 1765. This building houses the National School of Fine Arts in San Miguel de Allende, Mexico. The dance studio has vaulted ceilings, large windows looking out into a fountain filled vast courtyard, and a forgiving silky dance floor that measures its age in centuries.

One day almost two decades ago, in this majestic building, a student rolled into one of the full-length mirrors and it shattered. A falling shard sliced her calf. As you can imagine, this was a class stopper. The next week, someone warming up in the same spot of the room tweaked his knee. A week later, yet another person was injured, this time breaking a toe while simply walking across the same spot on the floor.

These three experiences so close together made me recall other incidents in this same location. In the geography of this studio, it appeared this spot was NOT a good place to dance. We began to pile our backpacks and clothing in this area to keep ourselves safe.

This observation set in motion my inquiry into how geographies of dance studios and the layout of a space, both visible and invisible, support or undermine our investigation and teaching of Contact Improvisation. (I talked about the geography of dance studios in "Initial Contact".)

Students in my classes are not explicitly aware of how this inquiry affects how I guide the group. This is one of various subterranean elements of my pedagogy.

I told the dance floor story to Natanja den Boeft, a Contact teacher from Holland. This took us into a conversation about teacher's secret scores, tools, and spices. We decided to co-facilitate a lab focusing on these "secret ingredients" to see what we could learn from each other. This was at ECITE (the European Contact Improvisation Teacher's Exchange, 2003) in Findhorn, Scotland. We titled the lab "The Shamanism of Teaching Contact Improvisation." I did a similar lab with Angela Dony, from Russia, at the teacher's gathering before the Freiburg Contact Festival (2015).

As I recall these labs and go through four decades of journals, I realize I have collected numerous notes about these secret pearls of transmitting Contact Improvisation. I've sprinkled them throughout part two of this book. I've saved some that I consider important for this concluding section. I feel some vulnerability in offering these. I hope you find some helpful in your own teaching.

The incomplete human

A son or daughter's self-esteem goes up when the parents

embrace the facets that are unformed and unresolved in the child. Our children don't, at some point, become "completed" human beings.

There is a courageous willingness needed to make room within the dance for the parts of ourselves and our partners that are unresolved. We as dancers are never "completed." How do we endure and even celebrate the unresolved fragments of ourselves?

Teaching from our wounds

Carl Jung, in speaking about the wounded healer archetype, says our biggest gift to the community comes from our wound.

My role in my family was to be the "constellater." I had to make sure everyone was connected to everyone else, or I would get, as they say, the shit end of the stick. I got skilled at knowing what everyone in the room was feeling and how they were connecting to – or disconnecting from – one another. This wound, this skill, has been invaluable for me as a teacher to constellate groups of students.

The raw and tender excavation of our wounds makes us more aware and articulate. This gives us tools for teaching that can never be taught in a class setting.

When the treasury is full and when the treasury is empty

When someone's interior treasury is full, people rush forward to present that person with gifts. When a person feels rich and least in need, people freely offer them reverence and appreciation.

Paradoxically, when the interior treasury is "wanting," people try to pilfer the little that remains. When a person most feels the hunger for acknowledgement, it doesn't come their way.

This can be vital information for a teacher. If you are feeling a lack of acknowledgement, how is your treasury? Is it time to dance more in non-teaching situations? Do you need to spend more time in stillness or in nature? Are you in need of more input from those people whose brilliance you respect?

A teacher with an overflowing treasury creates a communicable generosity in the group. This invites everyone's treasury to over-flow, and the room brims with dancers bestowing gifts on one another.

O ur responsibility when our students leave the studio

It is important to recognize the analgesic qualities of Contact Improvisation. Dancing can allow our personal struggles and existential ache to rest. This is a valuable state for receiving fresh information.

This dance form can also dislodge or strip people of their familiar self-identities. Old patterns and boundaries change. Once useful behaviors are no longer effective. This can be disorienting and frightening.

What is our responsibility as teachers when we bring people into this state? How do we ease people back into their everyday lives, without them experiencing a strong backlash? As teachers, we can help by keeping people connected to the companionship of sensation.

Retrieve parts of ourselves

How do you recognize when you are bordering on shamanic teaching? Using the word shamanic in this context can imply we are trying to retrieve parts of ourselves, possibly by invoking extra-ordinary states. It implies we are using the places in us or around us, where there is a gap into these coexistent domains.

If you have ever attended a birth or a death, you may have noticed when the light in the room changes. One way to sense we are near this ephemeral boundary is that a similar light appears around the edges of the studio and in the spaces between people.

You cannot will it into being. You can only prepare the ground.

Full dissolution while teaching

You are dancing. You have dissolved into the dance. There is no sense of you and other; there is ONLY the dance.

Slicing through this moment of sublime transparency, a blemish or knot appears. Your knee hurts, or you get irritated at your partner's insensitivity, or you judge yourself for losing the flow.

How do we draw a bigger circle here, so the present moment includes the blemish? How can we see the knots as part of the flow? How can we make the knots a facet of the transparency?

When we get bumped, yet again, from this state of dissolution, where do we find compassion for ourselves, the other, the dance, and keep the spirit of invitation alive?

T eaching while gob-smacked

When a person maintains a meditation or single-point practice for years and decades, they may develop "*siddhis*" or powers. In teaching Contact Improvisation over time, some people develop the *siddhi* of vulnerability. They speak in an open and naïve way. They start where they are and trust it will lead somewhere. Or as Munju Ravindra says, "*They hobble around gob-smacked by the beauty and despair of the world.*" This is mostly an unassailable place, a powerful place.

A spiritual impulse

A student once said from her wheelchair in a closing circle, "Contact Improvisation is a physical expression of a spiritual impulse."

If we accept that, to say "Yes" to one instance is to say yes to all of existence, then this form stems from a spiritual impulse.

P recious and rare moments for intention setting

The Northern California Contact Jam at Harbin Hot Springs is five days in a beautiful locale, with wonderful people and dancing as the main activity day and night.

During these events, we regularly hold "dream pools," where we sit in a circle and the participants put in their dreams and desires for the jam and for their lives.

At my eighteenth jam over New Years, I put in the desire that I would like to see people dancing Contact Improvisation full-out while nude. I thought, "Yep, that will never happen."

As we danced out the old year, a group of twelve created a count-down score for the moments leading to midnight. They each wore ten items of clothing and with every countdown – 10, 9, 8 etc. – they stripped off one piece of clothing until, at midnight, they were nude. To my delight, they had full-out, wild Contact dances.

My dream came to life!

That night, I realized I had almost always received the desires I had spoken into the dream pools over the years. I wondered why, with such a record of success, I had been speaking my small-time desires?

At the next jam, I spoke into the dream pool my desire to meet the woman who would be my partner for life and the mother of my children. Within a year, she appeared. And the following year, she attended the jam with me, pregnant with our son, Dylan.

That was two decades ago.

All around the world, I see dancers contributing their generosity to forming Contact communities. We can become alert in our time together to these precious moments for inten-tion setting, both individually and as a community. In these moments, with like-minded people, we inhabit both sides of the boundary, and our voices can be heard by the powers that be.

Embers in the Heart Conclusion

 Any time we risk really hearing someone, letting who they truly are

dance against the intimate core of our being, what we give that person

is the gift of themselves. When the space in us is an invitation,

we find things around us answering by coming alive. It is in the nature

of things that a beautiful opening inspires us to find something

of equal beauty to put within it.

– Charles Johnston "The Creative Imperative"

When the group constellates as a whole

There is a moment during class when everything changes. It's the moment the group constellates as a whole, it's the moment the teacher can leave off tracking the individuals and track the integrated group.

Sometimes, this constellation happens within minutes of a group gathering for the first time. Many groups take two or three meetings. For a handful, it never happens.

When a group constellates as a whole, you will notice a conspicuous change. Beforehand, when the class sits in a circle and the individuals speak, they address only the teacher. After the transition, they speak their observations and comments to the everyone.

To arrive at the constellation, several strategies and tools are helpful. Serious, focused work helps a group constellate, as do play and laughter. It can bond people to go so deeply into the details of sensation that people lose their normal narrative for a time.

One element that encourages this transition, I call embers in the heart. It is the place in the teacher where the smoke of excessive enthusiasm has burned away, and the coals are ready for sloweddown cooking.

This radiance can arise from a passionate engagement with the dance form. For some teachers, the coals ignite simply by the presence of students. The embers can emanate from where a person is most well-rounded and from where they are most wellwounded. And this may be the same place. What is cracked within us can lead us to the place of our gifts.

When we shift into the constellation, the embers in everybody's heart can get fanned and shimmer off one another. These shimmering embers allow each person to move beyond his or her selfdefinition. Each person gets to discover something concealed, and a spirit of invitation appears.

ACKNOWLEDGMENTS

Over the decades, people have stepped up as pillars of support in my attempts to wrangle my imaginings and ideas into language. They've helped me to clarify, specify, and get to the heart of the topic. Most importantly they keep insisting I put words onto the page the same way I speak them aloud.

My heartfelt gratitude for vital and straightforward feedback goes to:

Arye Bursztyn, Brad Stoller, Brenton Cheng, Carol Swann, Carolina Fernandez, Cynthia Williams, Daniel Halkin, David Koteen, Deborah Whitehurst, Dey Summer, Dharam Kaur Khalsa, Elise Knudson, Eszter Gal, James Schlesselman, Jenny Doell, Jenny Epstein Kessem, Jill Cooper, Julie Nelson, Kees Lemmens, Leandro Howlin, Leslie Cohen Rubury, Lisa Nelson, Melanie Hedland, Melanie Rios, Nancy Stark Smith, Nicola Visser, Peggy Dobreer, Pen Dale, Rhonda Morton, Sarah Carr, Sarah Jaffe, Stefanie Sherman, Steve Bryson, Sue Lauther, Susan Singer, Ulli Wittemann, and always, Liza Keogh.

(After 30 years of doing this, I know I've missed many who have helped along the way. If you are one, please remind me so I can add you to future versions of this list.)

martinkeogh.com

-
-
-
-
-
-
-
-
-
-
-
-
-
-

martinkeogh.com

92684150R00152

Made in the USA
Columbia, SC
02 April 2018